OVERWEIGHT or OBESE?

You Can Lose It

Dr. Richard Ng

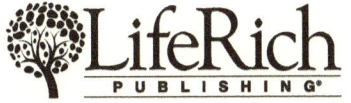

LifeRich
PUBLISHING®

LifeRich Publishing is a registered trademark of The Reader's Digest Association, Inc.

LifeRich Publishing books may be ordered through booksellers or by contacting:

LifeRich Publishing
1663 Liberty Drive
Bloomington, IN 47403
www.liferichpublishing.com
1 (888) 238-8637

Because of the dynamic nature of the Internet, any web addresses or links contained in this book may have changed since publication and may no longer be valid. The views expressed in this work are solely those of the author and do not necessarily reflect the views of the publisher, and the publisher hereby disclaims any responsibility for them.

Any people depicted in stock imagery provided by Thinkstock are models, and such images are being used for illustrative purposes only.
Certain stock imagery © Thinkstock.

ISBN: 978-1-4897-1147-2 (sc)
ISBN: 978-1-4897-1148-9 (hc)
ISBN: 978-1-4897-1146-5 (e)

Library of Congress Control Number: 2017903949

Print information available on the last page.

LifeRich Publishing rev. date: 03/17/2017

FOREWORD

Losing weight is not easy for most people, but losing weight and keeping it off is even harder. A Gallup survey published in February of 2016 showed that the obesity rate in the U.S. surged in 2015 to a new high of over 32 percent, an almost 7 percent point increase since 2008. This means an increase of about eight million adults in the U.S. who are dangerously overweight over a seven-year period, from 2008 to 2015.

It is not surprising that overweight and obese adults make up about 68 percent of the U.S. population. This statistic is based on Gallup's Body Mass Index calculations using self-reported survey data on height and weight. The statistics for children are not encouraging either, with 17 percent of those between 2 and 19 years old reported to be obese.

Obesity, undeniably, is fast becoming the top health problem in the U.S. We spend, both by the Government and the private sectors, hundreds of billions of dollars every year for the treatment of obesity-related conditions such as cardiovascular diseases, diabetes, hypertension, hyperlipidemia, as well as decreasing productivity due to lost time at work.

An analysis prepared in 2014 by the National Center for Weight and Wellness at George Washington University estimated the annual cost of obesity at $305.1 billion. This mind-boggling figure includes direst and non-direct medical services, workers productivity losses, disability issues and premature deaths. Unfortunately, this astounding costly trend seems to be climbing without any relief in sight.

A recent survey by the World Health Organization (WHO) of the most obese countries in the world, using the percentage of adults with a Body Mass Index (BMI) over 30. The normal range of BMI is between 18.5 and 24.99. Topping the obesity list is the Cook Islands where more than half of the population is obese. The U.S. is ranked somewhere in the middle of the list of 30 most obese nations.

According to the data from the American Medical Association, the Center for Disease Control and Prevention, State Departments of Health, and Statistic Brain Research Institute, the following U.S. cities have high adult obesity rates:

Memphis, Tennessee	34.9%
Nashville, Tennessee	34.5%
Detroit, Michigan	33.1%
New Orleans, Louisiana	32.4%
Oklahoma City, Oklahoma	32.1%
Indianapolis, Indiana	32.1%
Birmingham, Alabama	31.0%
Cleveland, Ohio	28.7%
Orlando, Florida	28.3%
Milwaukee, Wisconsin	28.3%
Las Vegas, Nevada	28.2%
Charlotte, North Carolina	28.0%

Tampa, Florida	28.0%
Providence, Rhode Island	28.0%
Hartford, Connecticut	27.7%
Houston, Texas	27.7%
Louisville, Kentucky	27.6%
Phoenix, Arizona	25.7%
Buffalo, New York	24.2%
Riverside, California	24.0%
Los Angeles, California	23.9%
New York City, New York	22.0%

Obesity has certainly reached an epidemic proportion in our country and deserves more of our attention, personally and nationally. A 2016 survey conducted by the American Society for Metabolic and Bariatric Surgery and the University of Chicago found that 81% of Americans now consider obesity to be the greatest health threat facing the country, tying it with cancer and putting it ahead of heart disease, diabetes, and mental illnesses. Weight loss business is a twenty billion dollar industry, if not more! However, there is no reason to lose hope because plenty of studies have shown that lasting weight loss is possible, not a myth.

CONTENTS

CHAPTER ONE

Problems with overweight and obesity

Most of us know that being fat, overweight or obese, is not good, and we hear about this all the time in social settings. Even parents often tell their children not to get fat. I am wondering how serious these parents are when giving advice to the children. I don't think most of the adults really understand and are aware of the significant problems that can be caused by overweight and obesity. Some of the problems may surprise you and hopefully you will be more enlightened to pursue a healthy journey to maintain a healthy weight. In this chapter, we are going to look at some of the major health problems related to overweight and obesity.

Obesity and hypertension.

First and foremost, obesity is considered one of the major causes for hypertension and this has been proven in many researches. According to the population studies, almost two-thirds of the people suffering from obesity are at risk of hypertension; hypertension is about twice as prevalent in the obese than the non-obese. The exact mechanism of how obesity causes hypertension is still unknown and many scientific data are still inconclusive at this time.

Hypertension, though treatable, is a major risk factor for heart disease and stroke. In the United States, nearly one of every three adults has high blood pressure. Hypertension accounts for approximately 38 million doctor visits annually, and it accounts for nearly 26,000 deaths in the U.S. This medical condition, also known as ' silent killer ', costs our country about $46 billion every year.

Many foods that are more likely to cause elevated blood pressure will generally lead to overweight and obesity. Many experts have found that diet can play a very important role in the treatment and control of high blood pressure.

If you are overweight or obese with hypertension, you need to avoid some of the foods and drinks described in the following:

- Bacons. They are loaded with heart-unhealthy fat and cholesterol plus a good dose of sodium. Together, they will put your blood pressure through the roof!

- French fries. They are loaded with saturated fat and hydrogenated (or trans) fats sometimes along with the salts. These can definitely increase your cholesterol and your risk of heart disease.

- Frozen pizzas. While you may find some healthy frozen pizzas with some difficulty, most of them can contain as much as 2,500 milligrams of sodium along with lots of carbohydrates and fat. They are fattening and bad for your blood pressure.

- American Chinese food. A common entrée such as beef and broccoli or Kung Bao chicken can contain almost 3,000 milligrams of sodium, not counting the soy sauce. This horrific load of salt can substantially raise your blood pressure and cause you to retain excess fluid. A double whammy for obesity and hypertension.

⌗ Cheese. It usually contains lots of sodium along with fat. Cheese lovers might want to cut consumption down, especially if you are obese and hypertensive.

⌗ Canned tomato sauce. In its natural form, tomatoes are one of the best foods with lots of nutrients. Commercially processed tomato sauce can contain a great deal of sodium, detrimental to your blood pressure.

⌗ Sauerkraut. It has many health benefits, but people with weight and blood pressure problems are advised to avoid it due to its high content of sodium, about 460 milligrams in one serving.

⌗ Red meat. An average serving size contains about 1,500 milligrams of sodium plus a lot of heart-unhealthy fat. You can enjoy your prime rib or sirloin steak once in a while; pick the lean meat which is grass-fed.

⌗ Pumpkin seeds. Despite their many health benefits, people with hypertension need to watch their intake because one small cup of pumpkin seeds will give you about 700 milligrams of sodium.

⌗ Pre-packaged noodles, commonly known as ramen. It contains a lot of salt, particularly in the small package of soup base. A typical package of ramen can have up to 1,600 milligrams of sodium.

⌗ Frozen pot pies. These are very convenient microwave food items, but each pie contains about 1,400 milligrams of sodium in addition to some of the bad fat.

⌗ Alcohol. Even though there are some health benefits associated with moderate drinking, which is being defined as one drink a day for women and up to two drinks a day for men, my advice to people who are overweight or obese, especially with a diagnosis of hypertension or pre-hypertension is abstinence because alcohol can aggravate blood pressure according to some studies. Of course, an occasional glass of red wine for your enjoyment socially or at home is perfectly acceptable.

☤ Deli meats. These include salami, turkey, chicken and others which are seemingly healthy. Please be reminded that they are processed meats with large amounts of sodium.

Obesity and heart disease.

Being obese puts you at a higher risk for heart disease because fatness is associated with a number of comorbidities including hypertension as already discussed briefly, dyslipidemia (increased levels of LDL cholesterol and triglycerides), impaired glucose tolerance and several forms of heart conditions.

As your BMIs increase, your risk of fatal and non-fatal heart disease increases. Congestive heart failure (CHF) is common in people with obesity and to some extent is related to systemic hypertension, even though many obese people can suffer from congestive heart failure in the absence of hypertension. CHF is characterized by abnormal left ventricular mass and function. At postmortem, sudden death of people with severe obesity was most frequently associated with CHF, severe coronary atherosclerosis (blockage of the coronary arteries) and pulmonary embolism (blood clots in the lungs).

Obesity and kidney stones.

Another relatively common medical problem encountered in people who are overweight or obese is kidney stones. Larger body size may result in increased urinary excretion of calcium, oxalate, and uric acid, thereby increasing the risk of kidney stones. This increased risk seems to be greater in women than men. These stones are made of salts, minerals and other substances, and when they are out of balance in the body, the risk of stone formation in the urine increases.

In one large study of 250,000 women and men, researchers found that, after adjusting for age, diet, fluid intake and the use of water pills (known as diuretics), obesity was strongly linked to kidney stone development. So, being obese or gaining weight may predispose you to developing painful kidney stones.

Obesity and diabetes.

Another very serious health problem associated with overweight and obesity is diabetes. In fact, the link between type-2 diabetes and obesity is so interdependent and strong that we have coined the term 'diabesity' for it.

Both insulin resistance and defective insulin secretion appear very early in obese people. Many studies have shown that an increase in overall fatness is specifically associated with insulin resistance, a cardinal sign of type-2 diabetes. Despite multiple risk factors for type-2 diabetes, the single best predictor is overweight or obesity.

Almost 90 percent of people living with type-2 diabetes are overweight or obese. The number of diabetes cases among American adults increased by a third during the 1990s, and more are expected. This striking, rapid increase in the occurrence of type-2 diabetes is mostly due to the growing number of obese people in the U.S.

Diabetes is a terrible medical condition, affecting all the systems and organs of your body with far-reaching complications. Its morbidity and comorbidities are beyond the scope of this book to cover. To reduce your risk of this awful disease, you must keep a healthy weight which is discussed in details in the following chapters.

Obesity and dementia.

Obesity can bring you brain problems also. According to one large recent study of more than 8,500 people over the age of 65 published in the journal Neurology, people who are obese in middle age, with a Body Mass Index of 30 or above, are at almost four times greater risk of developing dementias such as Alzheimer's disease in later life than people of normal weight.

Exactly how excess body weight can influence the degradation of the brain is not very clear. There can be many mechanisms, but we already know that higher body fat is associated with diabetes and cardiovascular disease, which are related to higher dementia risk. Anyway, growing scientific evidence suggests that controlling body weight and maintaining a healthy weight can reduce your risk of dementia.

Obesity and depression.

Data from the National Health and Nutrition Examination Surveys, 2005-2010, showed that 43 percent of adults with depression were obese, and adults with depression were more likely to be obese than adults without depression. Furthermore, the proportion of adults with obesity rose as the severity of depressive symptoms increased.

Depression can lead to overeating and weight gain; obesity can lead to overwhelming sadness. Researchers see the link between obesity and depression; there is an apparent weight-mental health connection. But, does depression cause obesity, or does obesity prompts depression? Medical experts are still trying to get to the bottom of the relationship so they can come up with effective treatments for both conditions.

Regardless of what is ahead in the medical-scientific agenda, it is in your best interest to lose weight and maintain a healthy body weight in order to decrease your risk of depression.

Obesity and Pleasure.

In a study published in the Journal of Neuroscience, an area of the brain called the striatum was less activated in women after they had gained weight. The striatum plays an important role in encoding the reward you get from eating certain foods such as those high in sugar that are associated with the release of dopamine in the brain, a chemical to experience pleasure. Being overweight or obese seems to be associated with this dulling effect which can lead a person to overeat in order to regain that sense of pleasure.

Obesity and vitamin D deficiency.

Obese men, women and children are 35% more likely to be vitamin D deficient than normal-weight people, according to a 2015 meta-analysis. The one possible explanation is given in a study published in 2000 in the Journal of Clinical Nutrition. The researchers found that obesity limits the body's ability to use the sunshine vitamin from both the sunlight and dietary sources, since fat cells hold on to the vitamins and don't release them efficiently.

Obesity and Neuromuscular function.

Studies of the elderly people find that obesity is associated with changes in brain activity that affect neuromuscular function, including making it harder to grasp. This can impair functions like opening a pill bottle for medications or gripping the railing of a staircase. The latter can certainly increase the risk of falling when the grip is not reliable. People with obesity and prediabetes have the propensity to develop polyneuropathy, according to a recent research conducted at the University of Michigan and published in the October 2016 issue of Journal of American Medical Association Neurology.

Obesity and sleep apnea.

Sleep apnea is common among obese people, especially those with the BMIs over 40, called morbid obesity. Sleep apnea is a dangerous and growing health problem in the U.S. It is undeniably and inextricably related to the obesity epidemic in our country.

The condition is caused by obstruction of the airway while asleep; loud snoring is its most benign form while the more serious sign is complete cessation of breathing. The low levels of oxygen in the blood can cause cardiac arrhythmia. These episodes of apnea causes frequent night-time awakening and non-restorative sleep. People often complain of morning headaches, fatigue, day-time sleepiness, listlessness and moodiness the next day.

Obese people tend to have larger tonsils and tongues, and larger neck circumferences, which can cause airway obstruction while sleeping. The size of the neck is generally a good predictor of sleep apnea risk. Obese men with a neck circumference of 17 inches or greater, and women with a neck circumference of 16 inches or greater are more likely to develop sleep apnea. With sleep deprivation and resultant hormone imbalances, these individuals with sleep apnea tend to eat mindlessly, creating a vicious cycle.

So, if you want to sleep better and breathe better, lose some weight. It is never too late and every pound counts.

Obesity and Sex Life.

From your body image to your hormonal balance, your weight can play an important factor in maintaining satisfying sexual experiences. Psychologically speaking, for most people, how you feel about your body is a big part of how you feel about having sex. Of course, there are other hangups everyone has that may contribute to what goes on in the bedroom.

In addition to the psychological aspect, overweight and obesity can create a host of problems, both physically and physiologically, like hormonal imbalance and erectile dysfunction. I am not here to say that obese and overweight people have poor sex life, but after reading this, you may find out hopefully how overweight and obesity can impact your sex life in ways you never realize.

For many individuals, overweight and obesity do correlate to lower levels of energy and motivation, limiting ability and/or desire.

Being overweight can sometimes make you focus on the negative about your body, not feeling sexy or wanted.

Men who are overweight or obese, experience a greater percentage of erectile dysfunction than men with normal weight. Research has shown that obesity lowers testosterone levels in men.

For men and women, higher levels of body fat means that you will have higher levels of a chemical called Sex Hormone Binding

Globulin, or SHBG. This chemical binds to the sex hormone testosterone which is present in both and women. When there is too much testosterone bound to SHBG and not enough available to stimulate desire, your libido will suffer.

Studies have found that obese and overweight men and women have decreased blood flow to their genitals because the extra weight caused their blood vessels to constrict or narrow. Sufficient blood flow is critical in order to reach an orgasm, and this is the basis of the prescription medications used to treat erectile dysfunction.

If your partner is overweight, he or she is most likely already stressed and beating himself or herself up. The best thing that you can do is to encourage him or her to be active, eating healthy, and showing your support in a positive way.

Obesity and early death

Recently, a large international study that included Harvard researchers links a higher BMI to a risk of early death. This should not be surprising considering the multiplicity of health issues and complications with obesity.

CHAPTER TWO

Obesity and the four common foods.

Obesity, which is fatness in layman's term, is the increase in the body fat and occurs in both the sexes. It can affect any age group. There are several factors which are associated with increasing the amount of body fat that results in obesity. These factors include genetic, metabolic, psychological, sedentary lifestyle, social and cultural, and high calorie nutrition. Weight gain occurs when you eat more calories than your body uses. Simply put, if the food you eat provides more calories than your body needs, the excess is converted to fat.

Considering the different factors causing obesity, the major reason in the U.S. is the foods that many Americans eat every day, which often contain a high number of empty calories. With all of the health problems related to obesity and overweight, obesity is no laughing matter. If you don't consider wisely the food you buy and eat, the world will soon be filled with people suffering from the problems of unhealthy weight.

There are four very common foods that cause obesity in the U.S. in my opinion, namely, sugar, white bread, potato chips, and fried chickens.

Sugar

It is the major culprit and should be on the top of the short list. First time ever, our Government, the U.S. Department of Agriculture (USDA) issued guidelines in 2015 and suggested limits of added sugar. It recommends that consumption of added sugar be no more than 10 percent of overall calories per day. For example, if you are eating 2,000 calories a day, that is about 50 grams for allotted sugar, or about 11 teaspoons.

But organizations including the American Heart Association and the World Health Organization recommend cutting the amount further; they say no more than 25 grams of added sugar a day is best for optimal health.

You really should look at sugar as a potential ' poison ', and from that perspective, you will become more mindful of it when you are eating and drinking. Many studies have shown that sugar consumption is the number one cause of unhealthy weight gain. Sugar is found in most of the processed foods, which means you are often consuming more than your recommended share but may not be aware of it. So, educate yourself and read the food labels to detect any hidden added sugars.

Do not become part of the unhealthy statistics which reveal that the average American in the U.S. consumes a whopping 130 pounds of added sugar annually! Most of us probably cannot deny that we all have sweet teeth and the taste buds for sweetness are sitting at the tip and front parts of our tongues.

There is sugar in the ketchup, and even in the French fries. All the added sugar has a priming effect on your body and brain. If you eat something sugary, you will want more sugar. Besides its addictive, potentially toxic properties, it has been linked to hyperactivity and emotional distress in teenagers, especially among those drinking four to five 12-oz cans of soft drinks every day.

Ironically, we were born with a love for sugar even though most people know that sugar is not good for you. You will not die if you have a couple of scoops of your favorite ice cream or your favorite donut or cookies, every now and then, and not on a regular basis. Just for your information, Americans consume about two billion gallons of ice cream a year, approximately twenty billion dollars in terms of expenditure by the consumers. This is astounding when you start to think of it. Having a treat can be a healthy pleasure in the right direction, as long as you can control it and are able to balance it with better foods and physical activity throughout the rest of the day, such as 30 to 40 minutes of walking.

Diets high in sugar cause insulin resistance, leading to type-2 diabetes. They also increase the levels of bad cholesterol (LDL) and triglycerides, and decrease the levels of good cholesterol (HDL), according to studies in the Journal of American Medical Association.

According to a 2013 study in the Journal of American heart Association, excess sugar is detrimental to your heart, both directly and indirectly.

Sugar is made up of glucose and fructose, and both are metabolized in the liver. When too much is consumed, the liver converts it to a lipid (fat). A 2008 study found that excess fructose consumption was linked to an increase in a condition called leptin resistance. Leptin is a hormone that tells you when you have had enough food. When leptin is dysfunctional under the influence of fructose, it leads to overeating of food and consequently obesity.

Sugar will give you calories, but not the full feeling that you get from other food like fiber, protein and fat. Thus, a diet high in sugar can lead to eating more calories than you need, which obviously can lead to weight gain.

Some studies have shown that sugar may be linked to the risk of cancer formation and may adversely affect cancer survival. When too much sugar is consumed, insulin does not work properly, and the body revolts, causing the cells to be more susceptible to cancer formation, according to a 2013 cancer research study.

There is alarming scientific evidence that sugar may affect the aging of your brain, resulting in impaired memory and cognitive decline, according to a 2012 study.

A major source of added sugar in the U.S. is the soda (soft drink). A recent study from the University of Texas found that those who drank soda, including diet soda were 65% more likely to be overweight than people who drank no soda. Diet soda contains artificial sweetener; many people choose diet soda over regular soda with the good intention NOT to gain weight. However, many scientific studies have shown that drinking diet soda is associated with weight gain.

The modern western diet, rich in fat and carbohydrates such as fructose, has been proposed to be an underlying cause of the increased prevalence of non-alcoholic fatty liver disease. Many studies have shown that sugar and alcohol have similar toxic effects on the liver.

Almost every cell in the body can break down glucose for energy; the only ones that can handle fructose are liver cells. When there is too much of it in the diet, it has potentially dangerous consequences for the liver. The liver uses fructose, a carbohydrate, to create fat, a process called lipogenesis. When the liver is given enough fructose, the tiny fat droplets begin to accumulate in liver cells. This buildup is called non-alcoholic fatty liver disease (NAFLD), because it looks just like what happens in the livers of people who drinks too much alcohol.

Virtually unknown before 1980, NAFLD now affects about 30 percent of adults in the U.S., and 70 to 80 percent of those who are diabetic or obese. With the excess sugar, the liver is under the effect of chronic inflammation. When this inflammation becomes severe, it can lead to cirrhosis, which is irreversible scarring, and eventual degeneration of liver function. Since NAFLD does not have any physical symptoms, you need blood tests and a liver biopsy for the diagnosis.

With all of the health problems associated with sugar, no wonder chronic overload of sugar may shorten your life. A 2013 study estimated that 180,000 deaths worldwide may be attributed to sweetened beverage consumption. The U.S. alone accounted for 25,000 deaths in 2010.

Hypertension is always known as a silent killer; I think it has found its competition: sugar is just as much a silent killer, if not worse. It is healthy and wise to cut back on both glucose and fructose. Fructose is the sugar from fruit, but don't do it by giving up fruit. Fruit is good for you and it is a minor source of fructose for most people. The major sources of fructose are refined sugar and high fructose syrup.

How about eating sweet, antioxidant-rich fruits? This sugar is not the same as the kind that is used in your ice cream and many other processed foods. You must look at the added sugar differently from the sugar in fruit, because in fruit you are getting so much more nutrition compared to refined sugar. You are getting free-radical-fighting antioxidants, vitamins, minerals, phytochemicals, water and fiber; these nutrients in fruit are all health boosters. Thus, the total package is what makes eating fruit so good for you. In fact, many studies have found that increased fruit consumption, regardless of the fruit's sugar content, is tied to lower body weight and a lower risk of obesity-related diseases.

For the sake of comparisons, I am going to list and rank some of popular fruits by their sugar content:

One cup of serving size	Sugar content
Cranberries	4.3 grams
Raspberries	5.4 grams
Blackberries	7.0 grams
Strawberries	7.4 grams
Watermelon	9.4 grams
Cantaloupe	9.4 grams
Nectarines	11.3 grams
Peach	12.9 grams
Apple	13.0 grams
Pear	13.7 grams
Honeydew melon	13.8 grams
Orange	14.0 grams
Blueberries	14.7 grams
Grapes	15.0 grams
Apricot	15.3 grams
Grapefruit	15.8 grams
Kiwi	16.2 grams
Pineapple	16.3 grams
Plum	16.4 grams
Sweet cherries	17.7 grams
Bananas	18.3 grams
Tangerines	20.6 grams
Mangoes	22.5 grams

Pomegranates	23.8 grams
Figs	29.3 grams

White bread

It is a staple food for many of us in the U.S. Actually, there are very few nutritional benefits from eating commercially prepared white bread. And at 80 Cal/slice, it is a bad deal for maintaining a healthy weight.

One of the most important nutritional issues when it comes to white bread is the carbohydrate content. Carbohydrates have received a bad reputation for some time. In general, the commercially prepared white bread is composed mainly of carbohydrates. On the one hand, carbohydrates are essential for good health, because they provide much of the energy needed to make it through the day. Many people think that in order to lose weight they need to cut out carbohydrates completely. But if you are trying to lose weight while you are working out, you need to maintain a good supply of glycogen for your muscles and brain by healthy carbohydrates.

However, the type of carbohydrate often plays an important part in determining the nutritional quality of the food. There are two classes of carbohydrates:

Complex carbohydrates, which are fiber-rich foods that contain vitamins, minerals and antioxidants. They are slow digesting and can help prevent many serious health conditions.

The other class is the simple carbohydrates which break down quickly in the body causing sugar spikes. They can actually lead to the increase of many health problems. White bread is mainly composed from simple carbohydrates, highly refined flour and rapidly absorbed as sugar, which have been found to be linked to increases in obesity and diabetes, and can even lead to the development of cardiovascular disease. Simple carbohydrates are also frequently found in baked goods and other highly processed foods.

According to a recent study at the European Congress on obesity, two or more slices of white bread a day can put people at a 40% higher risk of becoming overweight or obese. Commercial white bread generally contains a significant amount of fat due to the inclusion of eggs, butter and oil.

Furthermore, many brands of white bread contain additives which can be harmful to your health. If you like or must have bread in your diet, try whole-grain breads instead, which have fiber and more nutrients. The fiber takes the body longer to digest and may leave you feeling fuller for an extended period of time, thereby, curbing appetite for added food and calories.

Fried foods

Consumption of fried foods, most commonly fried chickens, French fries and hamburgers, is associated with general and central obesity, according to a large Spanish study.

During frying, food is totally or partially immersed in oil that is heated above 180 degrees Celsius. This process modifies both the food and the frying medium. In contact with the hot frying oil, food loses water and absorbs oil. Fried food also undergoes pyrolytical decomposition in the surface layers, resulting in the formation of heterocyclic amines. Furthermore, frying food absorbs degradation products of the frying oil such as polymers and polar compounds. These products have been associated with different types of cancer and hypertension.

A Spanish observational study of 34,000 adults confirmed that high intakes of fried foods are associated with general obesity and central body fat deposition. According to recent studies of 9,623 women in the Nurses' Health Study, of 6.379 men in the Health Professionals Follow-up Study, and of 21,426 women in the Women's Genome Health Study, the results clearly showed that regular consumption of fried foods was linked to higher BMIs. In addition, the studies found that the association between over-consumption of fried foods and obesity was particularly pronounced among people with a genetic predisposition to obesity. However, researchers observed that genetic risk of obesity could be mitigated by simply changing an eating habit.

French fries have very few nutritional benefits and are one of the guiltiest pleasures; eating French fries is one of the fastest ways to make you overweight in a short time. A small serving of French fries from popular fast-food chains has an average of 200 to 330 calories. But with the growing popularity of supersized fries, you can have up to 700 calories for a large serving. You are much better off eating real potatoes instead, and the health benefits are even greater with the skin.

Fried foods are typically served in restaurants and fast-food chains. They usually contain trans fat and saturated fat with many calories per serving. If you continue to include them in your diet, you are bound to develop plaques in your arteries that will lead to heart attack, stroke and premature death. Many studies have already confirmed the link between saturated fat and arterial clogging (plaques in the arteries).

Another unhealthy fried food is bacon. It is really bad news for the bacon lovers. Most of the bacon's calories come from fat including the saturated fat in bacon. Saturated fat is known to be harmful for your cardiovascular system, it can also cause inflammation that accelerates the aging process.

Potato chips are very popular among us, young and old, but they are a time bomb for your health. They are tempting because they are crispy and tasty, coming in different flavors for your taste buds. They are loaded with calories, fat and unhealthy amount of salt, a dangerous and terrible trio. One serving, which is about 15 to 20 pieces, contains at least 160 calories and 10 grams of fat. The fat includes trans fats which stimulate interleukin 6, an inflammation marker, increasing inflammation within your body. To top it off, potato chips contain acrylamide, a carcinogen that forms when it is fried at a high temperature.

The fast food chains are the primary providers of the fried foods in the U.S., even though some items on the menu are not bad from the nutritional standpoint. Today, American families spend over 60 cents of every food dollar on meals eaten away from home, oftentimes more than three to four times a week. It is well known that eating out may lead to excess calorie intake and increase the risk of obesity because of large portion sizes and increased energy density of foods.

Fast foods are typically:

- High in calories
- High in fat
- High in saturated fat and trans fat
- High in sugar
- High in simple carbohydrates
- High in salt (sodium)

Whether you have the 'obesity' gene or not, this is practically and mostly academic, it is wise and healthy to avoid or cut down your consumption of fried foods.

Pizza

On any given day, more than 40 million Americans will eat pizza. It is considered the most popular meal in the world, and certainly one of the favorites in the U.S.

Since it is so popular, does that mean it is good for you? Experts would argue that pizza is not really bad for your health, the problem is when and how you eat it.

According to the report released by the Department of Agriculture, 13 percent of the U.S. population consume pizza on any given day; this jumps to 22 percent among children and teenagers.

Pizza is the second leading source of calories for America's children. Every day, 1 in 5 or 20% of children eat pizza. Since pizza is usually low in nutrients and high in empty calories, it should come as no surprise that pizza is a big contributor to childhood obesity. The only higher source of calories in children comes from sweets, cookies and other sugar-rich snacks

In general, American men eat more pizza then women. Most of the time, pizza is bought from a fast food chain, or a local pizza restaurant, or frozen at a supermarket. Researchers at the European Medical Institute of Obesity suggest that eating pizza is one of the reasons why the U.S. has such high numbers of obesity cases.

Pizza was introduced in the U.S. at the beginning of the 20th century due to the influence of Italian immigration. Pizza can be a great source of nutrients in the American diet, especially when you make it at home with healthy ingredients. It is the commercially-prepared ones, which often are high in salts, carbohydrates and saturated fat, that I am concerned about.

As you know, most of the pizzas are consumed at night, sometimes late in the evenings. The latest research suggests that eating food high in saturated fat and carbohydrates at night can lead to an increase in body fat, thus contributing to obesity.

Rates of childhood overweight and obesity are on the rise, especially for minority children. Pizza should not be a part of the daily diet for anyone, children and adults. Childhood obesity is becoming a public health issue, requiring aggressive campaigns and initiatives by our Government so that this alarming trend can be controlled and reversed.

So, next time you are out with friends or family, resist serving yourself and the children pizzas, and give yourself and your kids a healthy meal instead.

CHAPTER THREE

Obesity and two common drinks

The two common beverages in the American society nowadays are alcohol and soda (regular and diet). From the nutritional standpoint, they are unhealthy, but they are so popular and ubiquitous. You find most restaurants serving alcohol and soda; those eateries that do not have the liquor license, they serve a lot of soft drinks, often with free refills.

You find local bars and taverns in every community, small or large, serving both alcohol and soda. You can buy alcoholic beverages and soda at all the airports, at all the hotels and resorts, and of course at all of the casinos. You can even find soda at all places of learning, including elementary and secondary schools, and colleges and universities. There are some government efforts to eliminate soft drinks, the sweet beverages from public schools, especially at the elementary and secondary levels. This is very commendable and a good healthy start.

Ironically, you can find soda at many, if not all, hospitals. Of course, many homes are stocked with beer and soda, which are on sale quite often in supermarkets and department stores. Many private parties at home, you can often find beer and soda, in addition to liquor. Almost all of the events held at banquet halls such as wedding, anniversaries, birthday celebration and so on, provide unlimited soft drinks and alcoholic beverages. There may be some limited alcoholic consumption when there is a cash-bar.

You easily see alcohol and soda everywhere in your daily life, and it is difficult not to notice their presence and many will eventually succumb to their temptation. The following will address the different health problems that are associated with their consumption, especially if your intake is on a regular basis. Hopefully, after you read this chapter, you will be able to eliminate soda from your diet or at least cut it down considerably, and drink alcohol mindfully with moderation. I am going to start with soda, regular and diet:

Sodas and diet sodas

These beverages including energy drinks are toxic sugars in disguise. Soda and diet soda, comparatively speaking, are very inexpensive; you can buy a case of 24 – 12oz cans for about four dollars and up to eight dollars, depending on the brands and time of sale. Almost all nutritionists and dieticians advise people to avoid soda and sugary drinks completely. Soda can become an addiction for some people similar to tobacco, alcohol and drugs; it feels good when you drink it, it can wreak havoc on your body long-term.

Many researchers have shown that they are directly linked to weight gain and all other diseases associated with it, from type-2 diabetes, heart disease and hypertension to cancer, dementia and infertility. According to a Gallup survey, there were fewer people consuming sugary drinks in 2014 compared to 2002, just a small decrease. The bad news is people might have replaced soda with booze, for better or worse?

Many people including children and young adults, the adolescents, still can't resist the sweet beverages. An average person in the U.S. drinks about 45 gallons of soda a year! This is an astounding quantity. A lot of researchers have already proven how unhealthy and toxic sugar is in the soda, which is essentially sugar-water. A recent study published in the American Journal of Public Health found that people who drank a lot of soda had shorter telomeres in the immune cells, meaning their risk of dying sooner is higher.

Telomeres are protective DNA units that are located at the ends of chromosomes, and the shorter they get, the more a person ages, increasing the risk of disease and early death. So, cutting out that good-for-nothing sugary drinks from your life will only offer you good things, by lengthening your telomeres as well as your life span, and improve your overall health.

A 2011 Harvard University study found that sugary beverages raise a person's blood pressure; another study in 2012 found that sugary drinks increased a person's risk of chronic heart disease. Other studies have shown that drinking a lot of soda can increase your risk of kidney disease and ultimately kidney failure.

Among the many health hazards, soda also destroys your teeth. In some extreme cases, drinking a lot of soda can leave your mouth as corroded as that of a methamphetamine abuser, according to a 2013 study. The citric acid in the soda erodes the tooth enamel, making it softer and more vulnerable to cavities and yellowing. You may not know that the phosphoric acid in the soda extracts calcium from the bones, increasing the risk of fractures due to weaker bones.

A recent study found that women who drank soda beverages had lower bone density in the hips. Thus, abstaining from soda will improve your bone health and lower your risk of osteoporosis. The less soda you drink, the more likely you may turn to milk or other calcium-fortified drinks.

Another potential alarming side-effect of soda is its negative impact on the brain. A study found that animals placed on a high-sugar diet had reduced amount of a chemical called brain-derived neurotrophic factor (BDNF), which in turn affected their ability to learn and remember things. Many other studies have also found a link between drinking a lot of soda and an increased risk of Alzheimer's disease or other types of dementia. This link showed an increased amount of plaque deposits in the brains of mice that were given sugary drinks – signals of Alzheimer's disease or other neurologic brain disorders.

Many soda cans, both regular and diet sodas, may contain Bisphenol-A, or BPA, which has been linked to an increased risk of cancer and impairment of the endocrine function. According to the Breast Cancer Fund, BPA can impair your hormonal system, increasing your risk for breast cancer, prostate cancer, metabolic disorders and even type-2 diabetes. BPA can also lower sex drive in men due to decreased testosterone levels and its estrogenic properties. One of the things BPA is known for is causing men to grow breasts by disrupting their hormones, a condition called gynecomastia.

Since we are on the subject of BPA, I feel it necessary to point out that BPA is also used in the plastic water bottles. You know it is important to stay hydrated, and many people are never seen without a bottle of water, you should consider trading your throw-away plastic bottles for the re-usable BPA-free variety. In 2014, the U.S. Government, the FDA, ended its authorization of the use of BPA in baby bottles and infant formula packaging. BPA is still a controversial topic, but it is better to be safe than sorry. I advise you to purchase typically items like tomatoes, in glass containers instead. If you are sticking with plastic containers, check for a recycle code of 3 or 7 on the bottom of the bottle that indicates the presence of BPA.

Many people switch to diet sodas with good intention of consuming less calories and trying to lose weight. Diet sodas taste the same as regular sodas because they have artificial sweeteners. They actually play tricks on your brain, which thinks the body is consuming more calories than it actually is, eventually leading to appetite problems. In the end, people end up eating more. You are much better off just drinking water or tea with slices of lemon. Another health problem with artificial sweeteners in diet soda is changing the gut microbes, increasing the risk of type-2 diabetes due to insulin resistance.

Artificial sweeteners or sugar substitutes are pure chemicals, and they include Saccharin, acesulfame potassium, sucralose, aspartame and neotame. Because they are devoid of sugar and calories, we tend to think we can consume as much of it as we want. To tell you the truth, they are in many ways worse and unhealthier than using real, natural sugar in this scenario.

Many studies have been done with the non-saccharin sweetener, aspartame, in diet sodas and found it to be a culprit for increased risk of insulin resistance and fatty liver disease. Experiments on rats with aspartame showed the increased risk of development of cancerous cells in different parts of the body. Some studies linked aspartame to a higher risk of multiple sclerosis while the Multiple Sclerosis Foundation and the FDA have rejected the association. Why risk it when diet sodas inherently can cause so many health problems anyway?

Aspartame has been linked to seizures; it also has been known to induce convulsions. This synthetic chemical can invade the blood-brain barrier, allowing the chemical to directly alter the brain's neurological function. It is believed that aspartame, which contains phenylalanine, can raise the levels of phenylalanine in the brain. It then reduces the production and flow of the neurotransmitters that protect against seizures.

One more thing you should be concerned about drinking regular and diet sodas is caramel coloring. In 2011, the non-profit Center for Science in the Public Interest petitioned the FDA to ban artificial coloring with caramel used to make Coke, Pepsi and other colas brown. The reason is two contaminants in the coloring, 2-methylimidazole and 4-methylimidazole have been found to cause cancer in animals. According to California's strict Proposition 65 list of chemicals known to cause cancer, just 16 micrograms per person per day of the 4-methylimidazole is enough to pose a cancer threat, and the popular brown colas, both diet and regular, contain 200 micrograms of this chemical per 20-oz bottle.

A few words about the sport drinks. Yes, they provide critical post-workout electrolytes like sodium and potassium, but they also serve up large doses of calories and sugar. In a typical 32-oz bottle of sports drink, there are 56 grams of sugar, which is more than a day's worth. Furthermore, some of those may have harmful additives and artificial coloring that have been linked to cancer and hyperactivity in children.

The popular energy drinks are packed with sugar, in addition to caffeine. Energy drinks have been linked to health issues like insomnia and cardiovascular disease. A recent study found that teens who drank energy beverages several times a day had later bedtimes, trouble sleeping and complaints of headaches. The high sugar level and its acidity of energy drinks can damage teeth and leave them more prone to stains that will age your smile. Moreover, their high caffeine and sodium content can lead to dehydration, especially if you are drinking them instead of water.

Alcoholic beverages

There are a few benefits coming from alcohol consumption in moderation. Women are not supposed to have more than one drink a day, and men are supposed to limit alcoholic intake to no more than two drinks a day. One drink or one serving of wine is 5 oz. with about half an ounce of alcohol. A 12-oz beer contains about half an ounce of alcohol. Spirit or liquor may vary in alcohol content. Personally, I advise my readers not to consume alcohol regularly, even in moderation. Essentially, you are walking a fine line between health and serious consequences. One drink or two occasionally or on special occasions are acceptable and should not pose any health problems. If you have some weight problem, it is best to avoid it.

Alcohol is a significant source of calories, even though it is still controversial whether moderate amounts of alcohol represent a risk factor for weight gain and obesity. Many people are not convinced that drinking alcohol is linked to obesity because research has so far produced inconsistent results. But, based on the energy-balance equation, regular alcohol consumption can lead to development of a positive energy balance, and thus weight gain.

Some research suggests that it is your pattern and amounts of drinking that affect your body mass index. A study of 37,000 drinkers found that BMI was linked to the number of drinks the subjects had on the day that they did drink. Researches from Yonsei University in Seoul, Korea, have confirmed a significant link between alcohol consumption and increased waist size and belly fat.

Furthermore, it is observed that drinking may stimulate overeating or eating mindlessly, particularly in social settings. Studies have shown that drinking can cause weight gain if:

- You drink heavily when you do drink
- You drink beer and liquor instead of wine
- And you have a tendency for weight gain to begin with.

Even though there is no conclusive causal relationship between alcohol consumption and obesity, there are, however, associations between alcohol and obesity, and these are clearly influenced by lifestyle, genetic and social factors.

Let us look at the problems which can be created by excessive alcohol consumption:

Diabetes. Besides causing you to pack on the pounds, it can increase your risk of diabetes even further, because it can cause sugar spikes with its carbohydrates and interfere with your body's production of insulin.

Infertility. It is a good idea to give yourself a break from the booze before you start trying to conceive. The research has shown convincing evidence that alcohol intake increases the risk of miscarriage, birth defects, and pre-term labor. In addition, the results of a Danish study confirm that even moderate alcohol consumption can lower a woman's chances of conception. Another Danish study of over 1,200 healthy men between 18 and 28 found that alcohol decreased both the motility and quality of their sperms.

Compromised Immune System. Most of your immune system is located in your intestinal tract. Heavy drinking has been linked to increased risk of leaky gut syndrome, in which micro perforations in your intestinal lining allow for particulate matter to leak out, potentially causing organ damage and other serious health issues. You will be more susceptible to illness because your gut bacteria are out of whack.

Bloating. With bacterial imbalance and increased inflammation of your gut, bloating with a puffy belly occurs as a result.

Breast cancer. Research suggests that women who have three or more drinks each week have a 15 percent greater chance of developing breast cancer than those who do not drink.

Gout. Alcohol can increase the levels of uric acid, promoting the development of uric acid crystals, leading to gout. These crystalline deposits can cause pain redness and inflammation, particularly in your joints; over time, this can compromise your mobility and increase your obesity-inducing inflammation.

Gastric acid imbalance. Alcohol has a tendency to increase your body's production of stomach acid, causing burning in the stomach, esophagus and throat. The development of gastro-esophageal reflux disorder can raise your risk of gastritis, ulcers and cancers.

Medication interactions. Alcohol can cause complications, sometimes dangerous, for the side-effects of certain medications, both OTC and prescriptions. These include OTC colds medicines such as Benadryl and sleep aids, prescription medications such as sleeping pills, anxiety medicines and certain antibiotics.

Hypertension and heart disease. The American Heart Association has confirmed that alcohol can cause a blood pressure spike, increasing your risk for hypertension. It is also a risk factor for heart attack and cardiomyopathy.

Stroke. With blood pressure spikes, this increases your risk of stroke. Researchers at Oulu University Central Hospital ad Helsinki University Central Hospital found that both regular alcohol consumption and instances of binge drinking are linked to increased risk of stroke.

Liver problems. The harmful effects of alcohol are well known. When your liver is damaged repeatedly over a period of time with excessive alcohol consumption, scar tissues begin to build, eventually impairing liver functions, resulting in a condition called cirrhosis. Many people with advanced cirrhosis, or end-stage liver disease will need liver transplants.

Kidney dysfunction. Alcohol gives your kidneys extra work with additional substances to filter out. Over time, it can cause kidney stones and other chronic renal disease.

Epilepsy. If you have a family history of epilepsy, it is wise and prudent to reduce your intake of alcohol. Research conducted by the Alcohol and Epilepsy Study Group shows that alcohol use increases your risk of seizures.

Cancer risks. There are many types of cancer directly related to the consumption of alcohol such as throat, stomach, esophagus and liver, according to many studies. Alcohol directly can cause your pancreas to become inflamed, putting you at risk for pancreatitis and pancreatic cancer.

Dementia. It is common knowledge that alcohol can impair short-term memory, but it also has long-term adverse effects on the brain. The results of a British study published in Age and Ageing suggests a significant link between alcohol consumption and dementia.

Dehydration. Alcohol is a diuretic, and in sufficient amount, it can cause dehydration including your brain, resulting in headaches and thirst. The dehydrating effect forces your body to draw water from other sources such as muscles, leaving you more prone to cramps and injury and less motivated to hit the gym.

Depression. Alcohol is a depressant of your Central Nervous System, and can deprive you of serotonin. As a result, it can exacerbate depressive symptoms in individuals with a diagnosis of depression. Due to lack of motivation, your muscles will get weaker under the influence of alcohol. According to research published in the Journal of Neurology, Neurosurgery and Psychiatry, alcohol can cause muscle atrophy and decreased motivation to exercise.

Neuropathy. Studies have shown that alcohol abuse can cause serious and painful nerve damage, further reducing your motivation to hit the gym or doing regular exercise.

Mental decline. Researchers from Sweden's Karolinska Institute found a significant link between binge drinking and lower IQ. Findings published in Alcoholism: Clinical and Experimental Research suggests that alcohol damages the parts of the brain associated with impulse control.

Sleep disruption. Alcohol can disrupt your body's natural REM sleep, meaning you are more likely to wake up throughout your sleep cycle and feel less rested in the morning.

With all the problems alcohol can cause you, it is not surprising for you to feel exhausted and de-motivated, often making it impossible for you to go about your day. Your body and mind will do just fine without alcohol; if you do drink, you need to do so mindfully to avoid havoc on your health.

When you are thirsty, think of water if you want to stay healthy. People often wonder how much water they should drink every day. Some health experts advise a minimum of eight 8-oz glasses of water a day; others recommend the daily consumption water to be calculated based on half of your body weight in ounces. For example, a 150-lb person should drink 75 ounces of water daily, unless you have a medical condition that restricts the quantity of water you should take in. Remember, your body may need more water depending on your activities and the temperature of your surroundings.

Having a glass of water with a piece of lemon in it first thing in the morning has a lot of health benefits. Don't worry, you can still get your caffeine fix immediately after. Our body is about 65 percent water, but many of us tend to take it for granted, and never realized how important and healthy water is. Here are some of the health benefits with water:

- A glass of water as the first thing in the morning helps cleanse residual acids from food in your esophagus during your sleep. At the same time, water also helps flush acids off your teeth.
- Drinking about 20 ounces of water can increase your metabolic rate by as much as 30 percent, according to a study in the Journal of Clinical Endocrinology and Metabolism.
- Drinking sufficient amount of water every day will help lose weight because water will make you feel a little bloat, suppressing your appetite. Do not worry about the possible discomfort with the bloat, which is very short-lived.
- Drinking water, especially first thing in the morning, is key to diluting the substances in your urine that can cause kidney stones to form.
- Dehydration is one of the common causes for headaches. Drinking enough water may help prevent a headache.
- Water helps flush toxins and wastes from your body. The more you urinate, the more toxins you flush out of your body. Some people might consider this a nuisance, but if you are serious about weight loss and good health, this is well worth it because you get to move more, meaning burning a few calories, while eliminating toxins and metabolic wastes from your body.
- Last but not least, water acts as a lubricant for your intestinal tract, keeping things moving to prevent constipation.

CHAPTER FOUR

Other causes of overweight and obesity

Undoubtedly, your eating habit plays a very important role in maintaining your healthy body weight, we are going to look at other causes of overweight and obesity which are not related to your food intake.

1. An inactive lifestyle. Most Americans are not very active, and personally, I think one of the culprits is the invention and evolution of automobiles. Many people spend hours every day in front of TVs and computers doing work, school assignments and leisure activities such as electronic games. In fact, just as few as two hours a day of TV watching time can lead to overweight and obesity, according to many studies.

   Automobiles compromise our walking or biking; our levels of physical demands decrease because of modern technologies and conveniences, and lack of or little physical education classes in school. Please be reminded that an inactive lifestyle can make you more likely to be overweight and obese. It can also raise your risk for cardiovascular disease, high blood pressure, diabetes, colon cancer and other serious health issues.

2. The lack of energy balance. This can lead to overweight and obesity. Energy balance is a simple equation: your energy IN should equal your energy OUT in order to maintain your body weight. Energy IN is the amount of energy or calories you get from food and drinks. Energy OUT is the amount of energy or calories your body uses for things like breathing, beating of your heart, digesting and being physically active. To keep your ideal body weight, the energy equation does not have to be the same on both sides every day. It is the balance over time that helps you maintain a healthy weight.

3. Medical conditions. Some hormonal problems may cause overweight and obesity, such as underactive thyroid glands (hypothyroidism), Cushing's Syndrome and polycystic ovarian syndrome (PCOS).

    With hypothyroidism, there is a decrease in the production of thyroid hormones, T3 and T4; your metabolism slows down, causing weight gain, weakness, fatigue and other symptoms. Cushing's Syndrome is due to the body's adrenal glands making too much cortisol, the stress hormone. People with this medical condition usually gain weight, have upper body obesity, a rounded face, fat deposit around the neck, and thin arms and legs. Women with polycystic ovarian syndrome often are obese, have excess hair growth, and reproductive problems and other health issues. All of the symptoms are caused by high levels of androgens present in PCOS.

4. Not eating regularly. Skipping meals, especially breakfast on a regular basis can increase your risk of overweight and obesity. It is important to start your day with a balanced,

healthy breakfast. An Imperial College, London study found that when people skipped breakfast, the reward center in the brain lit up when they were shown pictures of high-calorie foods. That means if you skip breakfast, you will be more tempted by unhealthy, calorie-dense foods and snacks later in the day.

Experts suggest that you should aim to eat about every four hours, but the timing will or may vary from person to person. Eating mindfully and regularly throughout the day keeps your metabolism running at full speed, prevents dips in your energy levels, keeps you alert, focused and motivated, and can help maintain your healthy weight.

If you have to skip a meal once in a while due to certain pressing circumstances, it is not the end of the world, and your body will adjust for the short term. But it is wise always to keep some healthy snacks around in case you have to skip a meal. Nevertheless, eating regularly is important for your health because skipping meals can have significant effects on your body and mind.

5. Genetics and family history. Studies have shown that your genes have a strong influence on your weight. Overweight and obesity tend to run in families, but I am not trying to find an excuse for you to eat mindlessly. Your chances of being overweight are greater if one or both of your parents are overweight or obese.

Children, more likely than not, adopt the habits of their parents. A child who has overweight parents who eat high calorie foods and are inactive will probably become overweight too. Studies have shown that a healthy eating lifestyle can mitigate the hereditary influence.

6. Psychological and emotional factors. Some people eat more than usual when they are bored, angry or stressed. Stress causes your body to increase the levels of cortisol, making you reach out for high –calorie comfort foods. Or, some people have difficulty controlling their appetite and desire for food, such as binge eating disorder (B.E.D.). Over time, this overeating will lead to weight gain and obesity.

According to data from the National Health and Nutrition Examination Surveys, 2005-2015, 43 percent of adults with depression were obese, and adults with depression were more likely to be obese than adults without depression. The proportion of adults with obesity increased as the severity of depressive symptoms increased. However, the study did not clarify whether depression or obesity occurred first because they were both measured at the same time.

Other studies have shown a bi-directional relationship, meaning obesity increases the risk of depression and depression increases the risk of obesity. This is a vicious cycle: depression can lead to overeating and weight gain, and obesity can lead to overwhelming sadness.

Studies published in the Journal of Obesity confirmed the adverse effects of obesity on mental health. Individuals suffering from depression are more likely to overeat or make poor food choices, and avoid exercising due to decrease or lack of motivation, becoming more sedentary and obese as a result. Obesity and depression are two major health problems among adolescents. Countries all over the world saw a marked increase in the prevalence of overweight and obese children and adolescents from 1980s to 1990s. In the U. S., the upward trend has continued into the 21st century. Currently, almost one-third of children and adolescents in the U. S. are either overweight or obese.

7. Medications. Certain medicines can slow your rate of metabolism, increase your appetite, or cause your body to retain water. Prednisone, a steroid, is notorious for causing weight gain due to fluid retention and increased appetite. Birth control pills can cause short-term weight gain due to fluid retention. Please check with your physician if you suspect that your prescription medications might be the cause of your weight gain.

8. Smoking. You may notice some weight gain when you stop smoking. There are two reasons for this: one reason is that food often tastes and smells better after smoking cessation. The other reason is because nicotine raises the rate of metabolism, so you burn fewer calories when you quit smoking. However, as you already know, smoking causes many serious health problems, including 480,000 related deaths a year, according to the American Lung Association. Smoking cessation is more important than some possible weight gain, which can offset by increased physical activities and healthy eating.

9. Age. When you get older, your rate of metabolism decreases, meaning your body burns less calories, leading to likely weight gain. You should decrease your calorie intake as you get older unless you can burn it with increased physical activities.

10. Lack of sleep. Many scientific studies have shown that lack of sleep increases the risk of obesity. People who are sleep-deprived seem to prefer eating foods that are higher in calories and carbohydrates, which can lead to overeating, weight gain and obesity. When you do not have sufficient sleep, between 7 to 8 hours every night, your hunger hormone, ghrelin, goes up and your full or satiety hormone,

leptin, goes down. Sleep deprivation also causes increase in your blood sugar levels, raising your risk for diabetes.

11. Too much eating out. Nowadays, American families cook and eat together less at home while spending over 60 cents out of every food dollar (or more) on meals eaten away from home. With the increased frequency of families eating out more than three or four nights a week, more and more consumers, adults and children, are being exposed to large portions of high-fat, high-sodium, high-sugar and high calorie foods. Although many consumers are aware of food labels and basic nutrition principals, they are unaware of how foods are prepared outside of the home. Food service establishments cooking methods include using highly processed foods, breading, deep-frying, added fats and sugar for flavoring. These attributes, along with larger portion sizes, can and will lead to overweight and obesity before you know it.

CHAPTER FIVE

N.E.A.T. and exercise

Many of us may not have the time to hit the gym for workout or regular intense workout; some may not have or want to spend money for paying a membership at the health clubs. The reasons are acceptable in most cases, but this should not prevent you from pursuing a healthy life to maintain a normal body weight. Weight loss is not a sprint, it is not even a marathon. It is the rest of your life.

There are a few activities in your daily life that can help burn calories and decrease the risk of weight gain if you just pay some attention. They do not require equipment or membership fee or much space around you. These are called non-exercise activity thermogenesis or NEAT for short.

Doing squats. Just be creative when you are doing your laundry; put the basket with clean laundry on the floor and stand up. Then for every article of clothing, you do a squat. For each load of laundry, you will probably do at least 25 to 30 squats.

Walking up and down the stairs. Most homes have either two stories or basements. If you have something to fetch or put away in the basement or upstairs, try to make it more than one trip; this will help tone up your muscle in the lower extremities and burn some calories. Just watch your steps on the staircase to avoid accidental injuries.

Lifting things. If you live in a home or an apartment, you will have things to move around sometimes including bags of groceries. At the airport, do not use the rollers for your carry-on luggage; it is for you to carry to burn some calories and strengthen your arm muscles. Lift something heavy without hurting yourself. When it comes to weight loss, more strength training equals more weight loss. Strength training helps burn calories and at the same time increase your muscle mass.

Fidgeting. Appropriate simple body movements instead of sitting still like in a meeting can burn up to 350 calories, according to a Mayo Clinic study which researched energy expenditure in different human posture and movement associated with the routines of daily life (the so-called non-exercise activity thermogenesis). Obesity occurs when energy intake exceeds energy expenditure. Another opportunity of NEAT is pacing while talking on the phone instead of sitting still talking for a long time.

The number of simple body movements you make each day, called NEAT, is associated more closely with body weight than is the daily amount of vigorous exercise, according to investigators from Mayo Clinic. They found that these simple body movements every day over time can affect your body weight significantly. Most of the people usually focus on the diet to control their body weight; but the energy expenditures of fidgeting cannot be ignored or under-estimated.

Singing and dancing. You will burn at least 140 calories in just 30 minutes, according to a study. This activity is also a mood booster according studies conducted in Sweden. Swedish researchers studied 112 teenage girls who were struggling with problems including neck and back aches, stress, anxiety and depression. Half of them attended weekly dance classes, while the other half did not. The girls who participated in the dance classes improved their mental health and reported a boost in mood-positive effect that lasted up to eight months after the classes ended.

Push-up. It is not a full workout, and it should be considered a NEAT. Pushups work your chest, shoulders and core (abdominal) muscles, improving your upper body strength and endurance levels. It does not require much floor space and it does not call for any equipment. You can do them anywhere and at any time; you can stop it anytime. I advise you not to do pushup immediately after eating when active digestive processes are going on.

Pushup is such a personal thing. It can be modified as needed. You can adjust the speed you perform a pushup; you can change the angle of your body, even the hand placement; and you can add more or less intensity.

Since you lift about 70 percent of your body weight during a pushup, it is a fairly good calorie burner. Strength training in general is good for weight loss because it increases your metabolic rate.

Walking. Humans have erect posture and are supposed to walk with their two legs as soon as they can master the skill. Walking is the easiest and cheapest ways for losing weight. It is the most recommended ' exercise ' for people with obesity or overweight. Personally, I consider walking a non-exercise activity and part of your activity of daily living (ADL). Walking can do a lot of great things for your body, especially when you are doing it regularly.

- It helps burn calories
- It can be done by most people

- It is relaxing and an ideal way to decrease your stress and re-set your mind
- It is safe, provided you are aware of the surroundings
- No training is needed
- No equipment is necessary other than some comfortable walking shoes
- Walking can save some money on gasoline when you are not using your car for short distance, at the same time it helps our environment
- It raises your heart rate and increases your circulation, thus improving your cardiovascular health
- It might reduce varicose veins according to studies at the Cleveland Clinic
- It will improve your digestion after a meal, getting things moving in the intestinal tract and keeping your blood sugar levels stable
- It will increase your good cholesterol, HDL
- It will help keeping your bones, joints and muscles strong and healthy
- You will reap the health benefits of the sunshine vitamin, D, if you are walking during the day
- It will improve your immune system to fight off diseases

I recommend setting a goal of 10,000 steps daily if you can, using a pedometer. Those who live in the northern parts of the U.S., walking can be done inside a shopping mall. Let me give you some idea about the number of calories burn just walking at a normal moderate pace:

If you are between 120 and 140 pounds and walking at a normal pace about 3 miles per hour:

15 minutes will burn 50 calories
30 minutes will burn 100 calories
One hour will burn 200 calories

While walking upstairs and downstairs at the same pace:

15 minutes will burn 120 calories
30 minutes will burn 240 calories
One hour will burn 300 calories

If you weigh between 140 and 160 pounds and walking at a normal pace about 3mph:

15 minutes will burn 60 calories
30 minutes will burn 112 calories
One hour will burn 225 calories

While walking upstairs and downstairs at the same pace:

15 minute will burn 130 calories
30 minutes will burn 275 calories
One hour will burn 545 calories

If your weight is between 160 and 180 pounds and walking at a normal moderate pace about 3mph:

15 minutes will burn 65 calories
30 minutes will burn 127 calories
One hour will burn 255 calories

While walking upstairs and downstairs at the same pace:

15 minutes will burn 155 calories
30 minute will burn 310 calories
One hour will burn 620 calories

Of course, if you can tolerate and do brisk walking at a faster pace about 4 to 5 miles per hour, your body will burn higher number of calories. The most commonly used equation to calculate that burn comes from the American College of Sports medicine. On a per pound basis, tall people burn fewer calories at any speed or covering any distance because they take fewer steps.

Laughing and chuckles. The body will burn 10 to 40 calories in 15 minutes of laughing and chuckling, according to Vanderbilt University researchers in ' Energy Expenditure of Genuine Laughter ' published in the International Journal of Obesity in 2006. So, watch a comedy or a funny show on TV; no wonder laughter is known as the best medicine.

Cleaning house and other housework. I know house cleaning is not a fun thing to do, but think of it as a calorie-burner, about 119 calories in 45 minutes, according to research. Besides the calorie burning benefit, it will give you some sense of accomplishment and your place of living will look better – mental health booster.

The Kaiser Foundation estimated that 56.6% of American women were overweight or obese as of 2011, a sharp increase from two decades ago. Many studies have suggested that modern American women spend less and less time in housework. Women's role in society has significantly changed, as full-time, often sedentary employment has replaced and decreased the amount of time women spent on housework.

Recent studies have found that the decline in physical activities, including housework is contributing to the increase in obesity in the U.S. Published in PLoS One, the study showed that women are doing far less housework in 2010 than they were in 1965, and this has led to a net reduction in energy expenditure of 360 calories a day. In 1965, women cooked, cleaned, and did laundry among other household chores, totally about 26 hours a week, while the amount of time spent in 2010 doing the same work declined to 13 hours.

I am not advocating or suggesting that women should go back in time doing more housework; in fact, housework should be shared by everyone in the household and it is a healthy thing to do. The working together within the household is also promoting and fostering inter-personal relationships. For your information, researchers observed that the amount of time women spent watching television, and later using the computer at home doubled from eight hours per week in 1965 to over 16 hours per week in 2010. For better health, we all have to increase our energy expenditures by increasing our physical activities.

Avoiding the elevators. If you work in the city, try to use the staircase instead of the elevator. Oftentimes, you will save some standing -waiting time while burning some calories. Do not forget that standing and stretching from your office chair every so often can also help burn calories and decrease stiffness.

Healthy parking. Value some minor changes in your lifestyle habits such as parking further away from the entrance of department stores and supermarkets, as long as the weather permits.

Swimming. I am including swimming in NEAT even though it can be considered an exercise, like walking. Here, I am not talking about competitive, high intensity swimming; I am referring to recreational, leisurely swimming, even just playing around in the pool, or on the beach by the ocean or lake and having fun.

Swimming is the best cardio, pulmonary and musculoskeletal physical activity (or exercise) one can do, in my opinion. It is a full-body work, using almost all of your major muscle groups. It increases heart rate, raising body temperature which in turn causes your body to burn calories. Personally, I think it is better than weight-bearing exercises such as running and jogging with impact and high intensity.

Swimming involves your upper and lower body work at the same time, while using the harmless resistance of the water. Studies have shown that swimming 30 to 40 minutes three to four times a week can reduce the risk of stroke, heart disease, type-2 diabetes, and lower bad cholesterol and blood pressure, while raising good cholesterol.

So, go and get some swimming lessons. Learning the proper techniques, body position and breathing skills will help you be more effective and efficient in the water, which will help you enjoy more, leading to weight loss. A study conducted by the University of Utah researchers found that swimming was just as effective as land-based exercise for weight loss.

Aquatic exercises or exercises in water (and you do not have to be a swimmer) can promote cardiopulmonary health, improve muscle strength, endurance and flexibility, and tone your body. Regardless of the aquatic activity you choose, your body weight in water is about 10% of your weight on land, thus putting less stress on bones, muscles and weight-bearing joints.

President Obama brought attention to an important issue for Americans in September, 2010 and declared September National Childhood Obesity Awareness Month. As you know, one third of all American children are overweight or obese. Childhood obesity, an alarming and ever-rising public health issue, has many health consequences; these include increased risk for diabetes, high cholesterol, high blood pressure, heart disease, sleep apnea, fatty liver disease and orthopedic problems.

Swimming is fun; overweight or obese children who reject the idea of exercise will be receptive to the idea of swimming or just playing in the water to begin with. There is less chance of injury in the pool due to low impact and proper supervision. There is no denying that it is an excellent activity to help fight against obesity and overweight, especially for the children.

For your information and comparisons, the following is a list of activities and their calorie burning on average in the first hour for a 200-pound person:

Hatha yoga	228 Cal
Slow walk	255 Cal
Bowling	273 Cal
Ballroom dancing	273 Cal
Tai chi	273 Cal
Canoeing	319 Cal
Slow, easy cycling	364 Cal
Volleyball	364 Cal
Power yoga	364 Cal
Golfing, carrying your club	391 Cal
Downhill skiing	391 Cal
Brisk walking	391 Cal
Low impact aerobics	455 Cal
Running on elliptical	455 Cal
Wright lifting	455 Cal
Baseball/softball	455 Cal
Water aerobics	501 Cal
Lap swimming	528 Cal
Hiking	546 Cal
Rowing on a machine (much better on a boat)	546 Cal
Water skiing	546 Cal
Cross country skiing	619 Cal
Backpacking	637 Cal
Ice skating	637 Cal

Racquetball	637 Cal
High impact aerobics	664 Cal
Roller blading	683 Cal
A game of basketball (recreational)	728 Cal
Flag football	728 Cal
Tennis, singles	728 Cal
Running at 5mph	755 Cal
Running uphill or upstairs	819 Cal
Vigorous swimming	892 Cal
Taekwondo	937 Cal
Jumping rope	1074 Cal
Running at 8mph	1074 Cal

I just can't say enough about the importance and numerous health benefits of physical activity and exercise, and I am not talking about the intensive workout. Exercise is essential for your body, but it also keeps your mind in tip-top shape. Let me briefly describe the benefits of exercise, hoping that you will realize you have everything to gain except for the pounds nobody wants.

- More energy. Even though you are using some energy to exercise, it actually gives you more get-up-and-go. When you exercise regularly, the fatigue disappears.

- Better mood. Exercise makes you feel good about yourself and happier because your body produces endorphins, the feel-good chemicals in the brain, when you exercise. The physical accomplishment, no matter how small, boosts your self-esteem and confidence.

- Better sleep. Doing regular exercise helps you fall asleep faster and sleep more soundly, and it does not matter when you do the exercise.

- Less stress. Exercise has a calming effect on your body and your brain. After exercise, the levels of adrenalin and cortisol drop, and anxiety and stress fade away.

- More productive. In one study, people who got moving in the middle of the day were much more productive when they went back to work. They were also happier and getting along better with their co-workers.

- Healthy weight. Exercise and diet work together to keep your healthy, whether you want to lose some inches around your waist or just avoid putting on extra pounds. Try to workout or do some routine physical activity for 20 to 30 minute a day, 4 to 5 times a week, and you will surprise yourself how easy and healthy you will feel.

- Longer life. Regular exercise can and will add years to your life, and that is true even if you are not a hard-core fitness buff. Just some exercise regularly can help you live longer than not exercising at all.

- Stronger bones and muscles. Exercise and physical activity can help ward off osteoporosis and protect your balance and coordination.

- Heart benefits. It is no secret that exercise and physical activity are great for your heart. It can lower your risk of heart disease, reduce levels of bad cholesterol, and control and even prevent high blood pressure.

⚖ Improving your joints. If you have arthritis, regular exercise can decrease your pain and stiffness, and make your daily activities easier. I highly recommend non-impact exercise like swimming; to make it enjoyable if you are a beginner, take some lessons.

⚖ Decreased cancer risk. According to some studies, regular exercise can cut your risk of some cancers including colon, breast, and lung. And people who have cancer experience better quality of life when they exercise.

Take a look at the exercise options and think about which one of these will fit your situation or you will like, and stick with it. Start slowly and incrementally without exhausting yourself. You can do as long as you want. Remember, you have everything to gain except the calories and cumbersome pounds.

If you are obese, you have a challenging job due to a significant amount to shed. Many obese people probably and mistakenly believe that they are too far gone to start any fitness program --- this is not true at all! Undoubtedly, what you eat is the most important aspect, accounting for 80% of your effort. The other 20%, of course, is how much you move. NEAT and regular exercise are always good for you because they can reduce your risk of heart disease, high blood pressure, hyperlipidemia (high cholesterol), diabetes, and improve your sleep and mood.

You need to start slowly and ease it in, to avoid ankle and knee injuries which are more common among obese exercisers. I suggest starting with low-impact, low-speed options such as walking on the treadmill or outside, swimming and dancing, for 15 to 20 minutes in the beginning. The length of the physical activity and exercise is not that important; making it a habit on a regular basis is actually more important. If you can do it on a daily basis, it is the most commendable.

Once you have become regular from the routine and repetitions, you can gradually increase the intensity to include some strength training such as weight lifting starting with a pair of 5-lb or 8-lb dumbbells or as tolerated. With some progress and consistency, you will be ready to set your short-term goal, like joining your first 5-K walk in two months. You don't have to get competitive with other people in a race; just outdo yourself as an incentive. Your only goal should be just to go a little bit further than you did the day before.

Remember that there are days you can go all the way, and there may be days you might have to struggle just to get to the next block. It is going to take time and consistency to reset your lifestyle habits and reverse the process. Your motivation will ebb and flow, and it is unrealistic to assume that you will be forever motivated to get up and exercise every day. The point is keep trying and do not give up.

CHAPTER SIX

Other ways to burn calories and lose weight

Starting a major weight loss journey can feel incredibly daunting, and losing weight does demand some life changes. After all, you need to burn 3,500 more calories than you take in to lose one pound. But if you cut 500 calories a day, you can lose one pound a week --- and it should be fairly painless.

Just think a minute, a simple thing that cuts, say, 400 to 500 calories a day has a multiplier effect; if it is something that you eat or do three to four times a week, you will cut about 1,500 calories. Over time, that is a lot of pounds burnt. So, focusing on one step at a time may actually be the key to helping you lose the weight for good.

Try to cut your calories gradually and progressively. To lose weight, you need to eat fewer calories than you burn and there is no other way around it. Aiming to cut 400 to 500 calories from your daily food intake when you start your journey. If, after a couple of months, you see yourself plateauing for two weeks or more, you might need to cut another 100 calories or increase your activity level.

Chewing rule. Experts advised fifteen to twenty chews for each mouthful. The exact count is not really that important; it is sensible and wholesome to chew your food completely before swallowing. This is the very first phase of digestion of your food. When you swallow your food too quickly, you are likely to swallow air which can cause abdominal bloating and flatulence. Eating slowly with complete chewing also allows you to feel fuller on less food. Research suggests that you can reduce what you eat at each meal by 100 to 120 calories this way.

Try the 80–20 rule. Americans are pretty much conditioned to keep eating until they are stuffed, and this is not promoting healthy weight. Residents of Okinawa, Japan, eat until they are 80% full; the island has the highest concentration of centenarians. No wonder that President Franklin said " Lessen thy meals, and lengthen thy life ".

Read the food labels. An educated consumer is the best care-taker of the living body. Look for whole grains and ' no added sugar ' or sugar less than 10 grams per serving. Also avoid MSG because it blocks the ' I am full ' hormone. Watch for saturated fats and their amount, and ditch trans fats.

Eat on a smaller plate. There is some evidence that the size of your dinner wares can influence how much you consume during a meal, based on some studies about optical illusion. Personally, I don't think this is that relevant as long as you have the ability and understanding of portion control.

Using red dinner plates. Some studies have shown that those who use red plates end up eating less compared to other plate colors. Sound quirky? Well, try it and you may have every ounce to lose!

Salad for lunch. Have a mixed salad with fruit and vegetables and nuts instead of a fat sandwich because the two slices of bread with mayo and other things added can tally up to 550 calories for your lunch before the drink.

Skip the happy hour. Alcohol is calorific and fattening. Skip your discounted liquor which can give you about 500 to 600 calories --- almost a meal's worth.

Switch to black coffee. If you typically have two cups of coffee a day with cream and sugar, this alone will add at least 500 calories to your body. Switch to black coffee which has less than 10 calories and reap all of the health benefits of caffeine.

Quench your thirst with water. Ditch the sodas, regular or diet and go for the water with slices of lemon. Consider 200 calories for each can of soda you skip, just two cans of soft drink save you at least 400 calories a day. Drinking more water can cut your food intake by at least 205 calories, according to a recent study published in the Journal of Human Nutrition and Dietetics.

Cook at home. Cooking your meals at home whenever you can. Of course, this requires some of your time and planning; it is worthwhile for the long term considering the health benefits with home cooking. A 2014 study found that people who cooked dinner at home consumed about 140 calories fewer than people who ordered in, dined out, or heated up pre-made meals. You can cut the calorie count further if you can prepare your own breakfast and lunch mindfully, that is at least a saving of 500 calories for your body.

A typical meal at an American, Chinese or Italian restaurant contains nearly 1,500 calories, a lot more than anyone needs at one meal. Do not be afraid or embarrassed to take some home instead of trying to finish it, especially when you are already satiated.

Putting down your fork. Putting your fork down between each mouthfuls at dinner will make you eat up to 300 fewer calories subconsciously, according to a study published in the Journal of the American Dietetic Association. For five sit-down meals a week, that is a saving of 1,500 calories, not counting other calorie burning activities might do for that week.

Avoid sleep deprivation. Try to get seven to eight hours of sleep every night. Many studies have shown that sleep deprivation not only slows your metabolic rate, but also increases your appetite for snacks and sweets. According to a study in the American Journal of Clinical Nutrition, people who slept four hours per night consumed 300 more calories than those who slept a normal amount of 7 to 8 hours. Well rested individuals are also more motivated to exercise, leading to more calorie-burning.

Choice of steaks. Unless you are vegetarians, most people would like to treat themselves with a piece of nice steak once in a while. Beef, especially grass-fed beef, has many nutritional values, but eating it every day is not advisable from a health perspective due to the high amount of saturated fats and the potentially harmful degradation products from high-temperature cooking. Swap your prime rib for a sirloin steak; a 16-oz prime rib has about 1,400 calories, while a piece of sirloin steak of the same size is only 700 calories.

Watch out for the freebies. Next time you are eating at your favorite Mexican restaurant, do not touch the chips and salsa. These deep-fried chips offer little nutritional benefit, a basket of them can pack in 600 calories or more before your meal even starts. Same with the butter and rolls in many American restaurants, and you need to resist the temptation of these so-called freebies with your meal.

Some nice restaurants offer olive oil for you to dip your bread in. Olive oil is healthy for cooking, but it is calorie-rich, especially as a condiment. If you are serious about losing weight, avoid the bread and olive oil altogether and you can save yourself up to 500 calories from that meal.

No food before bedtime. Once you are full and happy with your dinner, it is not a good idea to eat one or two hours before going to bed. A study in the British Journal of Nutrition reveals that eliminating night-time snacks help you consume 240 fewer calories a day. I am talking about this as a regular habit. I am sure we all have hungry feeling before bedtime once in a while; instead of turning and tossing in bed with hunger pain, some snacks high in clean protein and complex carbohydrates are acceptable and will not ruin your weight loss plans.

Gum chewing. Many people, especially among the younger ones, have the habit of chewing gum. Try to get the plain sugarless ones; if you chew a few pieces a day, it can add up 200 calories. One collateral benefit of gum chewing is: helping you remove ear wax if you have a buildup problem.

Stop multi-tasking while eating. Put away your phones and laptops during your lunch. People who used their phones tend not to remember their meal well, feel less full, and snack more in the afternoon, adding at least 200 calories more a day, according to a study in the American Journal of Clinical Nutrition.

Turning off the television. Eating in front of the TV can lead to overeating. According to researchers at the University of Birmingham in the United Kingdoms, distracted eating can increase the amount eaten by 10 percent on average.

Turning down the heat. The colder temperature may encourage fat burning. Many studies have supported this finding, including one published in the Journal of Clinical Investigation showing people who spent two hours a day for six weeks in a 63-degree room burned more energy than those who spent time in warmer temperatures. According to another study published in the journal Trends in Endocrinology and Metabolism, spending time in chilly temperatures can boost calorie burning 30 percent. Another study involving participants sleeping for four weeks in bedrooms with different temperatures: one bedroom at 75 degrees, one at a cool 66 degrees, and a very warm one at 81 degrees. After four weeks, the subjects sleeping in the cool room at 66 degrees had almost doubled their volumes of brown fat, meaning they lost the most belly fat.

Eating in front of mirror. I know that this is not always possible and available, either at home or in a restaurant. A study published in the Journal of the Association for Consumer Research found that when people watched themselves eat in a mirror, they chose healthier options and ate about 400 fewer calories on average.

Planning ahead. Use the freezer if you have to and plan ahead before going to bed. Look at your schedule for the next day and plan out what you are going to eat. This will help avoiding unhealthy decisions about food choices.

Be socially proactive. Try to meet new people and make new friends who enjoy living the healthy lifestyle you are now pursuing. You can also be socially proactive by finding a recreational sports you like, such as tennis; you not only burn more calories, but also more socially active. According to research published in the Journal of Human Nutrition and Dietetics, even after losing the weight, women who received social support from others are consistently more likely to maintain their weight loss compared to those who try to do it alone. The buddy system has positive influence on you; join a weight loss group on Facebook, reach out anonymously on Reddit or post all of your meals or workout on Instagram.

Dim your hunger. In a Cornell University study, researchers found that people who ate a meal under soft, warm lighting consumed 175 fewer calories than those who ate in a brightly lit environment.

Get a dog. If you are thinking about getting a pet, I suggest a dog unless you have some kind of allergy to animals. A dog makes good companion, and needs to be walked, sometimes, more than once a day. Walking your dog is a healthy activity; you may also get to know your neighbors better, thus widening your social circle and improving your mental health. All of these are beneficial in your weight loss journey.

Do not skip breakfast or any meals. Studies have shown healthy breakfast eaters are more likely to lose weight and reduce their waistline circumferences than those who skip their breakfasts. Regular breakfast eaters have better blood sugar control, healthier hunger hormone regulation, more energy for work and workout, and sharper cognitive function.

Skipping meals can lead to poor subsequent food choices, resulting in obesity. It may also contribute to muscle loss with decreased muscle mass. Less muscle, less calorie burning. According to a study published in Diabetes Technology and Therapeutics, the drop in blood sugar levels from skipping meals can cause moodiness and fatigue. So, it is important for you to start your day with a healthy breakfast.

Keeping bad foods at bay. Put unhealthy snacks out of reach and out of sight. The slight inconvenience will make you think twice about grabbing a handful of chips as you pass the pantry. The trick is supported by a Cornell University study where researchers found that when office assistants had a jar of candies on their desks they ate nine per day, and when the jar was moved out of reach, they only ate four.

Stepping on your scale. Nobody likes to step on a scale and anticipate the number staring back, but doing this everyday may help you reach your magic number by making you more conscious. According to a Cornell University study, frequent self-weighing and tracking results can help you lose weight and keep it off.

Most of us have a 9 to 5 jobs with you buttocks essentially glued to a chair all day. Your job takes up precious hours in the day that can otherwise be spent working out or preparing healthy meals. Your job can make you stressed for whatever reason; it can also disrupt your sleep pattern if you are required to work different shifts. Your job can keep you in the car commuting or on a plane for business travel. The hectic schedule and demand of your job can keep your scale from going down due to the sedentary lifestyle.

Here are some tips to help you burn a few calories, shed a few pounds off, or maintain your healthy weight with your job:

- Take the stairs instead of the elevators. According to a study at the University of New Mexico Health Sciences Center, a 150-pound person could lose at least six pounds a year just by climbing up two flights of stairs every day. Try to park your car far away from the entrance of your office building, and you will burn some calories from the walk. Doing this to burn calories every day will add up many pounds lost over time.

- Stand up to work. Offices in the U.S. are in a transition mode with many companies converting their cubicle setup to more open spaces. More and more offices have started to offer standing desks or desks that can vary from standing to sitting positions, knowing that sitting in a chair all day is linked to obesity, diabetes and cardiovascular disease.

- Prepare your own snacks and lunches for healthier eating at work, and avoid the order-in crowds which are prone to making unhealthy food choices. Make sure that your snacks and lunches are low in carbs and high in protein and fiber.

- Hydrate yourself at work with water and lemon, not soft drinks which are sugary. By sipping water all day, you will feel fuller for longer because water is a natural appetite suppressant.

- If your work has an exercise room, tone up with some weight lifting during your breaks. The muscles burn way more calories than fat tissues.

- If you travel for business often, you are bound to run into flight delay sometimes. Use the time to walk around the airport instead of sitting down because you will burn more calories this way.

- You can also make use of your down time at the airport doing High Intensity Interval Training (HIIT). With HIIT, you perform short bursts of an exercise at full throttle, then rest, then repeat. This kind of workout helps your body continue to burn calories even while you are sitting in the plane.

- Order some green tea. You know business travel can be stressful, and you don't need to make it worse for your body. When the flight attendant comes around to take orders for beverages, resist the urge for an alcoholic drink and ask for green tea instead, This will give you that warm, relaxing feeling without the extra calories.

- Catch up with your sleep in the plane. Be sure you bring eye-patches, neck pillow and ear plugs to help you sleep because sleeping in a crowded plane can be challenging. As you know, lack of sleep prevents your body from releasing those fat-burning hormones that are crucial for weight loss.

- Do not skip breakfast to go to work. Try to eat a breakfast with protein and fiber to keep you satiated most of the day and sugar levels stable to avoid cravings. A recent study at Yale University and the University of Connecticut found that those that skipped breakfast are more likely to be overweight than those that have breakfasts

- After work, avoid happy hours because you will find yourself unhappy in the long run with the added calories in alcoholic drinks.

- Looking for chores to do at home when you are not working instead of sitting in front of the TV or engrossing yourself in the computer for hours.

- For those who work night shifts, switch to green tea instead of coffee; the powerful antioxidants in green tea known as catechins literally melt the fat stored in your body and send you on your way to your goal weight.

- Wear your sunglasses when you leave your night shift. By keeping your eyes shaded, your melatonin levels will remain high and your body will be ready for sleep when you get home.

- Find some ways to do some exercise when your work is slow during your night shift. You can do pushups, meditation, yoga or weight lifting with dumb-bells which do not require much time. The dumbbells and the yoga mat can be kept in your locker easily. According to 2015 research from Harvard School of Public Health, following 10,500 healthy individuals over the course of 12 years, they found those who spent 20 minutes per day performing resistance exercise such as weight lifting were more successful in the fight against belly fat compared to those who spent equal time getting their cardio such as jogging and biking. Unlike cardio, which burns calories during the workout, strength training helps you burn calories even after you stop the workout.

People who practice yoga regularly tend to be more mindful about eating. Researchers think that the calm self-awareness developed through yoga may help people resist overeating.

- For a night-shift worker, one of the challenges is getting sufficient sleep during the day. A recent study in the Journal of Diabetes found that those who kept their bedrooms colder slept better and burned more fat than those that slept in warm temperature.

Many people probably do not realize that when you lose weight, your metabolism slows down because a smaller body requires fewer calories. Boosting your metabolism is the key for weight watchers. Some people inherit a speedy metabolism. Men tend to burn more calories than women, even at rest. For most of us, the metabolism slows down steadily after age 40. Although you cannot control your age, gender or genetics, there are other ways to improve your metabolism. Here are some ideas:

- Drinking black coffee. It will give you a short-term rise in your metabolic rate. Remember to resist the creamer and sugar.

- Remember green tea. It offers the combined benefits of caffeine and catechins, both can rev up the metabolism.

- Eating small meals with healthy snacks. When you eat large meals with many hours in between, your metabolism slows down between meals. Having some healthy snacks between small meals will keep your metabolism cranking to burn more calories over the course of a day. Some studies have shown that people who consume healthy snacks regularly eat less ar meal time.

- Build muscles. Your body constantly burns calories, even at rest when you are doing nothing. This resting metabolic rate is much higher in people with more muscles. Every pound of muscle uses about six calories a day just to sustain itself, while each pound of fat burns only two calories a day. The small difference can add up over time. After a session of strength training, muscles are activated all over your body, raising your average metabolic rate.

- Aerobic exercise may not help build muscles, but it does raise your metabolism. Include a few short bursts of jogging in your regular walking can burn more calories.

- Don't forget water because your body needs water to process calories. Any degree of dehydration slows down the metabolism. In one study, adults who drank eight or more glasses of water a day burned more calories than those who drank four. To stay hydrated and avoid overeating, drink a glass of water before every meal and snack.

- Spice up your meals. Spicy foods have natural chemicals that can kick your metabolism into a higher gear. Cooking your foods with some red or green chili pepper can boost your metabolic rate. Even though their effects are temporary, it you eat spicy foods often the benefits can add up.

꒐ More proteins. Your body burns more calories digesting protein than it does with fat or carbohydrate. Good sources of protein include lean beef, skinless chicken, fish, turkey, tofu, nuts, beans, eggs and low-fat dairy products.

CHAPTER SEVEN

Obesity and your cholesterol

People who are overweight or obese are more likely to have high cholesterol, called hypercholesterolemia, which is a risk factor for stroke and heart disease as well as diabetes. When you combine obesity and high cholesterol levels with high blood pressure and/ or high blood sugar, you have a perfect storm known as metabolic syndrome.

Unfortunately, the older you are, the more likely you will be diagnosed with metabolic syndrome, which currently affects one-third of all adults in the U.S. The diagnosis of metabolic syndrome include three or more of the following, according to the National Heart, Lungs and Blood Institute:

- Abdominal obesity with a waistline of 40 inches or more for men and 35 inches or more for women
- High triglyceride levels of 150 mg/dL or higher
- Low HDL cholesterol levels less than 40 mg/dL for men, and less than 50 mg/dL for women
- High blood pressure, greater than 135/85
- High blood sugar

Cholesterol is not fully water-soluble, so in order for it to be able to travel around the body in the blood stream, it must be contained within another particle known as lipoprotein, with a water-soluble exterior surface.

LDL cholesterol is a risk factor for conditions including heart attack, angina, peripheral vascular disease, stroke and TIA (mini stroke). In contrast, HDL cholesterol is associated with improved health outcomes including reduced risk of heart disease and stroke. Conditions, conditions that lead to elevated levels of LDL cholesterol tend to cause HDL cholesterol to decrease.

Diet and lifestyle are important factors in many cases of hypercholesterolemia. In particular, a diet high in saturated and trans fats is strongly associated with elevated levels of LDL cholesterol. Sources of saturated fats include animal-derived products such as dairy produce, cheese, butter, cream, meat, chocolate, palm oil and coconut oil. Ironically, consumption of foods rich in dietary cholesterol such as eggs, prawns and liver has little impact on the circulating levels of cholesterol in the blood in most people.

Trans fatty acids, commonly known as trans fats, also occur naturally in small amounts in beef and dairy products, but most dietary trans fats are industrially produced in a process known as hydrogenation, in which hydrogen is added to vegetable oil in order to make it more stable with longer shelf-life. The negative impact of trans fats is worse than that of saturated fats. Trans fats are also known to have inflammatory properties, contributing to insulin resistance, and are associated with increased risk of heart disease, diabetes and stroke.

People leading a sedentary lifestyle are at increased risk of hypercholesterolemia. Regular exercise along with smoking cessation are known to have a beneficial effect upon cholesterol levels by decreasing LDL and increasing HDL cholesterol.

Individuals with central or truncal obesity, where extra fat is deposited predominantly around the abdomen and upper body, are especially susceptible to hypercholesterolemia. This pattern of fat distribution is associated with increased levels of visceral fats.

High cholesterol does not just discriminate against the overweight and obese people; it can affect the young, old, seemingly healthy, infirm, active, or sedentary. Some with hypercholesterolemia maybe due to hereditary factor. Smoking cessation, regular exercise, and maintaining a healthy weight can help reducing the risk of developing high cholesterol, but the easiest solution to this problem starts on your plates. Research conducted at Baylor University Medical Center reveals that the right foods can be an effective way of preventing and treating high cholesterol.

Let us look at some of the foods which have a positive impact on your health by lowering cholesterol in your body:

- Oatmeal. Research conducted at the University Manitoba revealed that the beta-glucans in oatmeal lowered LDL cholesterol an average of 7%. The wholegrain will also fill you up. Its cholesterol-lowering properties have been well-documented in many other studies.

- Lemons. Research published in the Journal of Food Science reveals that lemon's main flavonoid compound, eriocitin, can decrease bad cholesterol in a high-fat diet.

- Chia seeds. Heart healthy and fiber-rich, these small things are a favorite for weight loss. Research conducted at the University of Tucson revealed that they increased HDL and lowered LDL cholesterol levels, in addition to their anti-inflammatory properties.

- Salmon. Its omega-3 fatty acids decreased LDL cholesterol by as much as 25%, according to a study in Japan, and research published in the American Journal of Clinical Nutrition. The same is true for mackerel, which is also high in omega-3s.

- Bananas. Research published in the British Journal of Nutrition found that the soluble and insoluble fiber in Bananas can help decrease LDL cholesterol.

- Pistachios. They are rich in healthy fat. A study of patients with high cholesterol published in the Journal of American College of Nutrition revealed that pistachios can decrease LDL and increase HDL cholesterol levels. Cashews and walnuts also have the same healthy impact on your cholesterol.

- Strawberries. Colored fruits rich in resveratrol like grapes and strawberries can help lower your bad cholesterol, according to a study published in the Journal of Molecular and Cellular Cardiology.

- Tomatoes. In addition to the many health benefits of this colorful plant, research conducted at Rome's Catholic University revealed that lycopene in tomatoes can decrease bad cholesterol levels.

- Okra. Research published in Nutrition reveals that it can help lower cholesterol. Many other studies also confirmed its blood-sugar lowering properties.

- Kale. An ideal veggie for shedding pounds. It is also great to fight heart disease, improve gut health and lower your cholesterol. The results of a Korean study indicates that regular consumption of kale is positively correlated with a reduction in bad cholesterol, even without weight loss.

- Peas. This childhood favorite has a healthy place in your adult life. A study conducted at St. Michael's Hospital reveals that green peas have a mitigating effect on cholesterol.

- Onion. This small vegetable is packed with antioxidants, and is proven to decrease bad cholesterol and help maintain a healthy LDL to HDL ratio, according to researchers from the University of Colorado at Boulders, Department of Ecology and Evolutionary Biology.

- Flaxseeds. A good and easy way to add heart-healthy omega-3s and fiber to your diet. These little soldiers are great cholesterol fighters, according to a study published in Nutrition and Metabolism.

- Dark chocolate. Researchers in Finland found that eating 75 grams of dark chocolate per day over a three-week period lowered LDL cholesterol while increasing levels of beneficial HDL cholesterol.

- Avocados. With their heart-healthy fats, studies at Penn State University have shown that avocados can lower cholesterol and decrease your risk of heart disease.

- Oranges. They contain many nutrients including vitamin C and fiber. A study conducted at the National Heart, Lung and Blood Institute revealed that men and women who regularly consumed fruit (including oranges) and vegetables can reduce their bad cholesterol levels significantly.

- Peanuts. A study conducted by researchers from Penn State and the University of Rochester revealed that foods high in monounsaturated fatty acids (MUFAs) like peanuts, can significantly reduce LDL cholesterol levels.

⚱ Apples. Regular consumption of apples can lower cholesterol by up to 29%, according to a French study conducted at the Universitie Paul Sabatier Institut de Physiologie. An apple a day may help keep the doctor away.

⚱ Black beans. A popular Mexican item for a reason. A study at Brazil's Universidade Federal de Vicosa reveals that rats in the lab which were fed a black bean diet had their blood cholesterol levels lowered by 35%. Beans, in general, are a great source of resistant starch, a type of slow-digesting insoluble fiber that feeds the good bacteria in your gut, triggering the production of the chemical butyrate, which encourages the body to burn fat as fuel and reduces fat-causing inflammation.

⚱ Spinach. A super-vegetable with many nutrients. A German study published in the Journal of Nutrition reveals that eating a diet rich in fruit and vegetables including spinach can lower your cholesterol significantly along with other positive, healthy changes.

⚱ Chickpeas. They are a rich source of fiber and can lower your risk of heart disease. According to a study published in the Annals of Nutrition and Metabolism, adding chickpeas to women's diet for a five-week period reduced LDL cholesterol considerably.

⚱ Cashews. They are a delicious, healthy snack with fantastic cardiac benefits. According to findings published in Nutrition Reviews, cashews can help prevent the risk of heart disease, decrease your risk of overall mortality, and lower your cholesterol levels.

⚱ Cinnamon. A wonderful spice for your life. Research published in Diabetes Care reveals that it can decrease bad cholesterol and reduce your overall risk of cardiovascular disease.

- Cauliflower. This cruciferous vegetable can help you fight cholesterol when consumed on a regular basis, especially in raw form.

- Green tea. One of the best, if not the best, beverage on earth. It will lower your body weight and LDL cholesterol at the same time, thanks to a compound found in tea, called epigallocatechin. It has also been documented as a longevity promotor.

- Hibiscus tea. Similar to green tea, ideal for weight loss and reduction of cholesterol. According to research published in the Journal of Science, Food and Agriculture, it can help lower your cholesterol levels and body weight significantly when consumed regularly.

- Blueberries. You cannot find any reason not to enjoy them. Research published in the British Journal of Nutrition reveals that foods rich in phytosterols, like blueberries, are very effective in lowering LDL cholesterol.

- Amaranth. These nutty grains are excellent for weight loss and reduction of cholesterol, according to a report published in Lipids in Health and Disease.

- Almonds. Commonly available and inexpensive, almonds are rich in monounsaturated fatty acids, MUFAs, which can help decrease your risk of heart disease and the levels of bad cholesterol, LDL, according to research published in JAMA Internal Medicine.

⚱ Shellfish. Shellfish like crabs without the butter, can help weight loss as well as reduce your bad cholesterol, according to a study conducted at the University of Auckland.

⚱ Lentils. Consuming legumes like lentil is a great way for vegetarians to get plenty of protein. They are also good for lowering cholesterol. According to researchers from Tulane University and Arizona State University Polytechnic, regular consumption of lentils can have a positive impact on your cholesterol.

⚱ Apricots. Research published in the American Journal of Clinical Nutrition reveals that fruits rich in beta-carotene, like apricots, can help lower cholesterol.

⚱ Bell peppers. A rich source of beta-carotene, like apricots, and they can help improve good cholesterol levels, according to a study conducted at the University of Michigan, Ann Arbor, Michigan.

⚱ Jalapenos. Research published in Open Heart reveals that the capsaicin in the hot peppers can decrease cholesterol, if you can handle the burn.

⚱ Brussels sprouts. They are powerful, aggressive cholesterol fighters. The results of a Japanese study reveals sulforaphane in Brussels sprouts can lower your cholesterol significantly, reducing your risk of heart disease and stroke.

⚱ Red grapefruit. A super fruit for weight loss and cholesterol reduction. According to studies at the Hebrew University Hadassah Medical School, red grapefruit can lower cholesterol, as well as having beneficial effects on heart health and blood sugar levels. They are rich in phytochemicals, bioactive compounds that recent research discovered, can stimulate the production of a hormone called adipopectin, which is involved in the breakdown of body fat. A study published in the journal Metabolism found that those who ate grapefruits for six weeks lost a full inch off their waistlines.

- Coconut. Either drinking the tasty water or using the oil for cooking, coconut can lower LDL and increase HDL cholesterol levels, according to research results in Sri Lanka.

- Walnuts. A great addition to your salad or snack list, they are packed with beneficial monounsaturated fatty acids. MUFAs. Studies conducted at the University of California, San Diego, showed that they can reduce bad cholesterol and the risk of heart disease.

- Pumpkin seeds. A healthy, delicious snack to have around you to help reduce your body weight and cholesterol levels.

- Alfalfa sprouts. Another cholesterol buster. Research conducted at the Indiana University School of Medicine reveals that they can help lower LDL cholesterol levels. Just wash them thoroughly before eating.

- Garlic. It has been gaining more popularity for medicinal use due to its many potential health benefits. Research conducted at Liverpool John Moore University School of Bimolecular Sciences reveals that garlic can reduce risk of heart disease while lowering the total cholesterol.

- Olive oil. An important and popular ingredient in the Middle East. Results of the Lyon Diet Heart Study finds that the Mediterranean diets rich in olive oil could be the answer to the heart disease epidemic, thanks to its cholesterol lowering properties and preventive effects against cardiovascular disease.

- Mushrooms. This humble plant has amazing health benefits. Research conducted at Memorial Sloan-Kettering Cancer Center's Department of Medicine reveals that mushroom can help fight cholesterol and certain types of cancer.

- Barley. According to studies published by the Food and Agriculture Association of the United Nations, barley is a great, natural way to lower your cholesterol.

- Brazil nuts. Their cholesterol fighting power is amazing, in addition to their other health benefits, according to a study published in Nutrition and Metabolism

- Dandelion greens. It is always good to add dark green veggies to your diet. You will not only receive all of the important nutrients for your body, but also have the benefits of lowered cholesterol levels, according to research conducted at the University of Maryland Medical College.

This is only a partial list of the foods which can help you reduce your body weight and lower your cholesterol. Just keep an open mind and be proactive and persistent, and you will get to where you want to be. Science has proven that the way you feel about yourself is inextricably intertwined with what you are eating.

CHAPTER EIGHT

Obesity and Belly Fat

Something many of us have in common: the belly fat; to be more medically correct, it should be called visceral fat. People with the belly fat or excess fat deposit around their midsection, even though their body weights may be within normal limits based on BMIs, are considered to have central or abdominal obesity. Not only does belly fat make it difficult to zip up your pants or jeans, it also increases your risk of cardiovascular disease, high blood pressure, type-2 diabetes, and premature death.

Belly fat is not a joke, seriously; it is more deadly than all the excess fat underneath your skin in your hips, legs and arms, called general obesity. We know that obesity is not healthy, and can cause heart disease, type-2 diabetes, hypertension and other health problems. However, there is growing evidence that abdominal obesity can be much worse than general obesity. Unfortunately, your age can be a factor to increase the risk of belly fat, because aging, in general, causes a decrease in muscle mass and an increase in fat content. Post-menopausal women have an added disadvantage due to diminishing levels of estrogen physiologically.

Central obesity is defined as waist circumference 40 inches or more in men and 35 inches or more in women. Modern medical technologies with computerized tomography (CT) and Magnetic Resonance Imaging (MRI) have made it possible to separate the fat located inside the abdominal cavity from the subcutaneous fat beneath the skin.

A recent study shows that thin people who are centrally obese are at greater health risk than people who are overweight or obese based on BMI. The results of the study are published in the Annals of Internal Medicine. In other words, an individual can be centrally obese and have normal BMI and that person is at a greater risk for many serious health problems.

This significant study involved over 15,000 U.S. adults and found that normal-weight people carrying excess fat around the midsection were twice as likely to die compared with people who were overweight or obese according to BMI. Researchers postulated that central obesity is associated with an increased accumulation of visceral fat, which is stored around the internal organs such as liver, pancreas and intestines. This visceral fat is more harmful than the fat beneath the skin-- called subcutaneous fat.

Visceral fat also leads to an increase of leptin, the ' satiety ' hormone that tells the brain when you are full. The constantly elevated amount of leptin is similar to insulin resistance – the leptin resistance. So your brain never shuts off, and the people with central obesity and visceral fat, as a result, overeating and bringing in more sugar and more insulin. What a vicious cycle!

Having a large amount of belly fat, based on many studies, increases your risk of:

- Cardiovascular disease
- Insulin resistance and type-2 diabetes

- Colorectal cancer
- Sleep disorders including sleep apnea
- Premature death from any cause
- Hypertension

Let us look at some of the things that can make you gain, not just general fat, but belly fat in particular:

- Excessive alcohol, including wine, beer and liquor.

- Sugary foods and beverage, a major culprit as explained in other chapter of this book.

- Fruit juice. Even the unsweetened one contains a lot of sugar, in particular, fructose, which causes insulin resistance and promotes belly fat.

- Trans fats. Notorious and dangerous, and a must to avoid.

- Fried foods. They include the popular chickens and fish, and are usually loaded with saturated fat, calories, sodium, and sometimes, trans fat. These foods are definitely belly fat promotors; eat them once in a great while if you really like them so that you do not feel deprived.

- Processed, fast foods. Usually, they contain lots of calories, sugar, salt and unhealthy fat, a sad and dangerous combination for abdominal and general obesity.

- Pizzas. They are loaded with calories, saturated fat and sodium, and will give you a pot-belly in a short time if you eat it often enough.

- Chips and fries. They have a lot of bad fats, both saturated and trans, sodium and calories. Stay away from them if you want to get rid of your belly fat.

- Milk shakes. An occasional treat is acceptable because most of them come with bad fats, many calories and sugar.

- A low protein diet. When you have a high protein diet, you will feel full and satisfied longer; your metabolism will speed up with a spontaneous reduction in calories. Several large studies suggest that people who consume the highest amount of protein in their diets are the least likely to have excess belly fat. When your protein intake is low, your levels of Neuropeptide Y (NPY) increase, leading to overeating and promoting belly fat.

- A low fiber diet. Fiber plays an important role in controlling your weight. In a study of 1,114 men and women, soluble fiber was found to be associated with abdominal fat reduction. For each 10 grams increase in soluble fiber, there was a 3.7% decrease in belly fat accumulation. One large study found that high fiber whole grains were associated with reduced abdominal fat, while refined grains were linked to increased abdominal fat.

- Cortisol and stress. Stress increases the levels of cortisol, which often leads to weight gain, especially around the abdominal region. Stress itself can also trigger poor eating habits.

- Imbalance of gut bacteria. The bacteria in your gut are collectively known as your gut flora, or microbiome. When there is an imbalance with less beneficial bacteria, this can promote weight gain including abdominal obesity, according to some research.

- Menopause. This is the time when women's estrogen levels drop dramatically, causing fat accumulation in the abdomen, rather than on the hips and thighs.

- Genetics. The tendency to store fat in the midsection of your body is partly influenced by your genes inherited. In 2014, researchers identified three new genes associated with increased waist to hip ratio and abdominal obesity.

- Not moving enough. Inactivity should be a no-brainer for obesity, especially abdominal obesity. In one study published in the International Journal of Obesity, researchers found that three weeks of structured long walks significantly reduced cholesterol levels and accumulation of belly fat. So, get moving and you will be healthier and looking better.

- Lack of sleep. Many studies have linked sleep deprivation with weight gain, which often includes abdominal area. One large study followed over 68,000 women for 16 years and found that those who slept five hours or less per night were 32% more likely to gain significant weight than those who slept at least 7 hours per night. The weight gain and sleep problems can often lead to sleep apnea. In one study, researchers found that obese men with sleep apnea had more abdominal fat than obese men without sleep disorders.

- Skipping meals. This is a bad idea because it will increase the chance of your binge eating later in the day. It will also put your body in a catabolic state, meaning it will start to break down lean muscle for energy and store fat.

- Not brushing your teeth after meal. A study of more than 1,400 people found that participants who brushed their teeth after each meal weighed less than the people who did not.

⚱ Not drinking enough water. According to a recent study, drinking 16oz of water before each meal can lead to weight loss because water helps to increase satiety, resulting in weight loss. Hunger and thirst can be confusing, and very often people will look for food to eat when they are actually thirsty. Even if you have a craving for food, thinking that you are hungry, a glass of water with a piece of lemon is not a bad choice.

Forget about the ' quick fix '. Cosmetic surgery cannot get rid of the negative effects of belly fat. Liposuction does not reach inside the abdominal wall, so it can't undo the harmful visceral fat.

There are many fat-busting nutrients already found in food, and they are powerful tools for weight loss:

⚱ Magnesium. It is an important mineral involved in over 300 biochemical processes in your body, such as muscle contraction and protein synthesis. It helps boost lipolysis, a process in which your body releases fat from where it is stored. Higher intake of magnesium is associated with decreased levels of sugar and insulin, according to a study published in the Journal of Nutrition. Increased levels of sugar and insulin are linked to fat storage and weight gain.

Sources: red pepper, strawberries, orange, kale, etc.

⚱ Arginine. This amino acid is one of the most powerful weapon for weight loss. Researchers found that administering arginine to obese women over 12 weeks resulted in a 3-inch reduction in waist size and a 6.5 pound average weight loss, according to a recent study published in the Journal of Dietary Supplements.

Sources: Tofu, eggs, grass-fed beef, peanut and walnuts.

🍸 Choline. This special B vitamin turns off the fat genes to decrease fat storage around your liver. Studies have shown that dieters who eat eggs for breakfast, lose weight faster because they are less hungry for the day.

Sources: Egg yolk, lean meat, shrimp and collard greens.

🍸 Potassium. It can help flatten your belly in two ways: it is critical in muscle recovery after a workout and it helps the body flush out water and sodium to reduce bloating. It is also important in maintaining healthy heart and kidney functions. Most of the Americans do not consume adequate potassium, according to the findings of University of Illinois researchers.

Sources: bananas, avocados, nuts and leafy green vegetables.

🍸 Omega-3 fatty acids. They are heart-healthy fats, and unfortunately, many Americans do not eat enough fresh fish for this important nutrient. They help decrease levels of triglyceride and blood pressure; they also promote weight loss by decreasing inflammation.

Sources: fatty dish like salmon, walnuts, chia seeds and flaxseeds.

🍸 Leucine. Another important amino acid for protein synthesis, which helps build muscle mass of your body. According to studies conducted at the University of Illinois, people ate high-leucine diets lost more weight and body fat than those with a low-leucine diets.

Sources: chicken breast without the skin, eggs, tofu, fish, beef and pork.

⚖ Resistant starch. They are also known as slow carbs. This nutrient passes through your small intestines without being digested quickly, feeding the healthy gut bacteria and helping you feel fuller and longer while burning fat.

Sources: oats, lentils, peas, bananas and chilled potatoes.

⚖ MUFA. It stands for monounsaturated fatty acids. These fats are good for the heart; they also increase satiety and prevent storage of belly fat. A study in Nutrition Journal found that participants who ate half an avocado with lunch reported a 40% decreased desire to eat for hours afterward. Avocados are rich in oleic acid, a MUFA.

Sources: Avocados, grass-fed beef, extra virgin olive oil, coconut oil and dark chocolate.

⚖ Calcium. It is known for bone health; but it is also important for cardiac function. Calcium, in addition, can help your body burn more calories and store less fat. Your insulin needs it to work properly.

Sources: Dairy products.

⚖ Vitamin C. A powerful antioxidant proven in many studies to help people cope with stressful situations. Stress causes increased levels of cortisol, which tends to make people opting for bad food choices, according to a study in the American Journal of Clinical Nutrition. The study also found that levels of cortisol and blood pressure decrease rapidly in anxious participants given vitamin C supplements.

Sources: citrus fruits and many dark, leafy green vegetables.

- Tryptophan. This amino acid is a precursor to serotonin, which gets converted into melatonin to promote sleep. Adequate sleep is important for weight loss according to many scientific studies. In order to have better motivation to exercise and build up muscle mass and burn calories, your body needs time to rest and recover.

  Sources: eggs, cheese, milk, pineapples, bananas, tofu, sunflower seeds and turkey.

- Zinc. This trace element is known for prostate health in men. Zinc deficiency is also associated with a weakened immune system and fatigue. It is necessary for the production of stomach acid, which helps break down the fats and protein into energy. Low levels of zinc can lead to low energy levels, prompting you to eat more.

  Sources: oysters, beef, lentils, chickpeas, quinoa and turkey meat without skin.

- Selenium. It is critical for proper thyroid function. Many people who have hypothyroidism tend to have deficiencies in selenium and exhibit a slowed metabolism and weight gain.

  Sources: Brazil nuts, tuna, shrimp, cod and poultry.

- B vitamins. They are important in energy conversion and metabolism of the body. Studies have shown that deficiencies of B vitamins, particularly B1 (thiamine) and B12, can lead to overweight and obesity.

  Sources: Beets, beans, sunflower seeds, spinach, yogurt, grass-fed beef, eggs and mushroom.

✠ EGCG. It stands for epigallocatechin gallate, an antioxidant found almost exclusively in green tea. It enhances lipolysis (breakdown of fat) and blocks adipogenesis (formation of new fat cells), and boosts thermogenesis (production of heat through burned calories). According to a large study of 1,100 people over a 10-year period, Taiwanese researchers found that those who drank tea regularly had nearly 20% less body fat than those who did not.

Sources: green tea

✠ Vitamin D. Aside from its many well-publicized health benefits, this sunshine vitamin has an important role in weight loss. The combination of calcium and vitamin D is essential to keep your muscles and bones healthy. A 2012 study found that supplementation with vitamin D was associated with a 7% decrease in fat. Another study from the University of Minnesota found a relationship between higher levels of vitamin D and fat loss, particularly in the belly area.

Sources: Fish, mushroom, fortified orange juice, milk, egg yolk, cod liver oil, tofu, caviar and pork.

The following is a list of foods, commonly available, that will help you lose fat, especially around your abdomen:

✠ Kimchi. This fermented cabbage is a good source of many vitamins including A, B and C. It contains plenty of good probiotics that aid digestion. A recent study in the Proceedings of the National Academy of Science found maintaining healthy bacteria in your gut can improve the intestinal lining, which in turn, decrease abdominal fat.

- Lentils. These little things are loaded with protein and fiber per serving to keep you full and satisfied for hours. They are also a great source of fat-burning resistant starch.

- Oatmeal. A terrific source of resistant starch, helping to boost your metabolism, burn fat and improve gut health. They are a near-perfect weight loss tool because they keep you feel fuller thanks to their slow-digesting fibers which prevent spikes in blood sugar. The fibers can also help decrease bad cholesterol levels.

- Pine nuts. Research has shown that the fatty acids in them can increase satiety hormones to make you feeling full. They are also packed with vitamin B1 and manganese, a mineral that aids your body metabolizing carbohydrates and protein.

- Potatoes. They are a good source of resistant starch; eating them in moderation can help your body burn fat. On the European Journal of Clinical Nutrition index, potatoes rank number one.

- Popcorn. Not the kind you get from the theaters. The plain popcorn is loaded with fiber and protein, and light and airy, easily filling you up.

- Red wine. According to some studies, people who drank wine in moderation have smaller waists and less abdominal fat than those who drank mainly liquor. Other studies show that one glass of red wine can increase your body's calorie burning up to 90 minutes.

- Salmon. This fish is loaded with monounsaturated and polyunsaturated fatty acids. A 2001 study found that participants who ate more salmon lost an average of nine pounds in the short study period than those who ate a low-fat diet and gained an average of six pounds.

⏳ Green tea. There is absolutely nothing bad about drinking green tea. Drinking green tea will keep you away from other unhealthy beverages. It is a weight loss elixior with catechins, a group of antioxidants with proven anti-inflammatory and anti-cancer properties. One particular catechin, known as EGCG (epigallocatechin gallate) blocks the formation of new fat cells while simultaneously boosts lipolysis, the process of breaking down stored fat, according to a study published in the Journal of Nutrition and Metabolism. So, drink some tea and lose some belly fat.

⏳ Kale. A superfood for your belly fat. The rich fiber of this dark, leafy green veggie can keep you feeling full while its other nutrients can turn off genes for belly fat.

⏳ Grapefruit. This is a fat-burning superfood. Eating half a grapefruit before each meal could help you lose up to a pound a week, according to a study. Another study published in the journal Metabolism found that participants who ate half a grapefruit before meals shrunk their waists up to an inch in only six weeks. Grapefruit is also 90% water which can fill you up, acting as a natural appetite suppressant.

⏳ Almonds. An inexpensive source of MUFA and PUFA, healthy fats. They help lower cholesterol and keep you slim. Almonds have fewer calories per serving than most other variety of nuts. According to a study in the International Journal of Obesity, people who added a daily serving of almonds lost more weight than those who didn't.

⏳ Apples. This colorful food contains pectin that helps slow digestion and promotes feeling of fullness. Studies have shown that eating a whole apple with your meal, as opposed to apple juice, is a natural appetite suppressant. Apples are also a great source of many antioxidants, vitamin C and fiber.

- Avocados. This superfood is packed with MUFAs, potassium, magnesium, folate, vitamin C and E. According to one study, people who regularly consume avocados weigh less and have smaller waistlines than those who do not.

- Cinnamon. This wonderful thermogenic spice contains powerful antioxidants called polyphenols, which can help ward off weight gain and belly fat, according to some studies. Sprinkle some of it onto your coffee instead of sugar to lose some fat.

- Eggs. Have a protein-rich breakfast with this healthy, inexpensive food. In a study, half the participants were fed bagels while the other half ate eggs. The egg group was found to have a lower response to ghrelin (the hunger hormone) were less hungry three hours later and consumed fewer calories for the next 24 hours. The egg yolk contains choline, a B vitamin that is essential for cell functioning as well as a compound that turns off the genes that cause your body to store fat around your liver.

- Pumpkin seeds. They are a rich source of fiber and protein, and along with zinc and potassium, they are favorites for people who are interested in weight loss.

- Oysters. They are a great source of zinc that works with the hormone leptin to regulate appetite. Studies have shown that overweight people tend to have lower levels of zinc than the thinner folks. A study published in the journal of Life Science found that taking zinc supplements could increase leptin production in obese men by 142%! As a bonus: oysters increase your libido and can improve erectile dysfunction for better sex, which is a calorie burning activity.

- Raspberries. Like other colored berries, they are nature's weight-loss pills. They are loaded with fiber to boost satiety. Their polyphenols have been shown to decrease formation of fat cells and zap abdominal fat. A recent American Journal of Clinical Nutrition study of more than 200,000 people found that a higher consumption of fruits with anthocyanins found in blueberries and other colored berries was associated with a low risk of type-2 diabetes and obesity.

- Cauliflowers. This food has very low calories, about 25 per cup, but it is loaded with filling fiber along with many good nutrients like potassium, vitamin C, K and B6 to help weight loss. To avoid bloating like broccoli, steam it instead of eating it raw.

- Whole grains. A Tufts University study found that participants who ate three or more servings per day (oats, quinoa, brown rice, and wheat) had 10% less belly fat than people who ate the same amount of calories from refined carbs (white bread, rice and pasta). There is no question regarding the health benefits of their soluble and insoluble fiber.

- Coconut oil. A study in the journal Pharmacology found that just consuming two tablespoons per day reduced waist circumference by an average of 1.1 inch. Its unique medium-chain triglycerides, unlike the long-chain fatty acids found in animal sources of saturated fat, does not seem to increase cholesterol.

- Sunflower seeds. These small things are packed with healthy, filling fiber. Along with their fat-busting magnesium, sunflower seeds are excellent snacks to get rid of your belly fat.

- Bananas. Known for potassium, but they also a good source of resistant starch, which is important for weight loss. Your body digests slowly and helps you feel full for longer while at the same time promotes your liver to switch to fat-burning mode.

- Vinegar. Very low in calorie, so do not be afraid of using it if you are trying to lose weight. A 2009 Japanese study found that the acetic acid in vinegar could increase feelings of satiety and prevent the accumulation of body fat. In another study in Bioscience, Biotechnology and Biochemistry, researchers found that study participants given apple cider vinegar over a 12-week period lost more weight, body fat and inches from their middle than participants that were given a placebo,

- Spinach. This dark, leafy green is rich in iron, folic acid, vitamin K and C, lutein and antioxidants. It also contains magnesium, which can help decrease blood sugar and insulin levels, promoting weight loss and reducing fat deposit.

- Sweet potatoes. They are a good source of slimming resistant starch which promotes the feelings of satiety. They are naturally sweet but low in calories.

- Greek yogurt. Its thick, creamy texture with abundant protein is very satiating. Studies have shown that the acids produced during yogurt fermentation could also help increase feeling of fullness, promoting weight loss.

- Chia seeds. A great snack for people who are serious about weight loss including the belly fat. They are packed with fiber, and a good source of omega-3s, calcium, potassium and magnesium, all of which are good fighters against obesity and overweight.

⌛ Coffee. In moderation, the caffeine in coffee can speed up your metabolism and help your body burn more calories. A study in Physiology and Behavior found that the average metabolic rate of people who drank regular coffee was 16% higher than those who drank decaf. Just try to avoid sugar and cream, which can offset any health benefits of your coffee.

The powerful combos for weight loss:

Sometimes, two is better than one, and the combination can also make your food tastier and easier to stick to. Each has its own nutrients and work together synergistically to help you keep hunger at bay, stay full longer and burn more fat and calories. For example:

⌛ Pistachios and apple. This is a good mid-day snack if you need it. The combination offer protein, healthy fats and fiber to fend off hunger. Pistachios are one of the lowest-calorie nuts with many health benefits.

⌛ Steak and broccoli. Do not be afraid to enjoy your steaks once in a while, as long as you choose the lean ones. Beef is rich in protein and iron, which your body utilizes to make red blood cells and carries oxygen, giving you more energy. Broccoli makes an excellent combination with beef with its powerful source of vitamin C and fiber, along with other nutrients.

⌛ Oatmeal and walnuts. This is a powerful combination for healthy weight loss. Oatmeal provides you with plenty of fiber which slows your digestion and takes up space in your stomach. Walnuts, besides their heart-healthy fat, add more fiber plus satisfying protein.

- Bean and vegetable soup. This weight-busting delight is a good addition to your lunch or dinner. Studies have shown that people who started their meals with healthy soup ate 20% fewer calories than those who did not. Beans like chickpeas or black beans can give you more staying power because of their high contents of protein and fiber.

- Green tea and lemon. Instead of ordering a soft drink, get a cup of green tea with lemon slices. Lemon provides you with the famous vitamin C and soothing aroma, while the antioxidant-packed green tea can help your body burn more calories and fat with its catechins.

- Yogurt and berries. Make it a colorful combo with either blueberries or raspberries which provide your body with fiber to keep you satisfied. Research has shown that calcium and vitamin D are good for burning fat.

- Chicken and Cayenne pepper. Skinless chicken breast serves up to 30 grams of protein for very few calories, a good deal for the weight watchers. Spice it up with Cayenne pepper or your other favorites like garlic or ginger to boost calorie burning.

- Scrambled eggs with green pepper and black beans. According to the studies published in the journal of the American College of Nutrition, people who ate eggs for breakfasts, consumed 22% fewer calories at lunch. Black beans and peppers make it more filling, thanks to a double dose of fiber, a real winner in your weight-loss marathon.

⏳ Dark chocolate and almonds. For sweet or chocolate lovers trying to lose weight, this is a safe combo. With its low sugar content, dark chocolate can be combined with the high-protein almonds as an attractive duel. This combination will keep your blood sugar levels steady and can keep you satisfied longer.

⏳ Salmon and sweet potato. This can be a wonderful lunch or dinner for the conscientious weight watchers. Fish is often called a brain food, but it is also good for your waist line due to its protein. Adding the naturally sweet potato in baked form gives you a filling sensation with only 112 calories in a typical five-inch long serving.

The above are only a few delicious but powerful combos for your fight against excess body weight, and you will be amazed and happy by the encouraging results with your motivation and perseverance. Of course, you can always design your own healthy food combinations for your personal taste and flavor.

CHAPTER NINE

Obesity, cravings and the brain

Why is it so difficult for obese people to lose weight despite the social stigma and health consequences such as high blood pressure, type-2 diabetes, cardiovascular disease, arthritis and even cancer, even though they have the desire to shed pounds? One of the main reasons scientifically is because certain types of food are addictive!

'Just say no ' is not that simple and easy, because there are specific biological mechanisms that drive addictive behavior. We live in a country of rich resources with democracy and freedom, our government and food industry both advocate more personal responsibility when it comes to fighting the obesity epidemic and its associated diseases.

Some nutritional experts posit that there is no good food or bad food, and it is all about a matter of balance and portion control. This is partially true in many aspects; new discoveries in science have proven that commercialized, processed foods (usually sugar-, fat-, and salt-laden) are biologically addictive

Let us put a big plate of broccoli or apple slices on the kitchen counter for the sake of demonstration. Do you know of anyone who would binge on the broccoli or apples? On the other hand, if you replace them with potato chips or cookies, the results may be very different.

More and more studies are suggesting that food made with fats, sugar and salt can be addictive, especially when combined with additives in discreet ways that food industry will not fully share or make public. Unfortunately, many people are biologically wired to crave these foods and eat as much of them as possible, a lot more than planned.

What is food craving? It is the all-consuming desire to look for and eat certain foods. In a study from Tufts University, 91% of women in the study said they experienced strong cravings for foods. Will power is not the answer. These urges are fueled by feel-good brain chemicals such as dopamine, released when you eat these types of foods, which gives you a rush of euphoria.

Cravings are characterized by intense desires typically relating to the anticipation of consuming pleasure-producing substances such as food. The word ' crave ' is derived from the Old English ' crafian ', meaning to beg. Nowadays, it is often linked to excessive pattern of substance abuse in the realm of psychiatry.

When you are stressed out or under pressure, your body releases the hormone cortisol, which signals your brain to seek out rewards such as comfort foods loaded with sugar and fat. This is the classic brain conditioning. Food cravings behave like waves; they escalate, crest and then disappear. Try not to give in to cravings which will ruin your weight loss efforts, and wait it out with whatever distractions you may have or find, such as listening to your favorite music, talking to your friends on your phone, reading some interesting articles in magazines or newspapers, watching news on the news channels, window shopping or simply just taking a walk.

Uncontrolled food cravings can become addictive, similar to chemical dependency and alcoholism. Food addiction is characterized by:

- Eating certain foods a lot more than intended, without the ability of portion control.

- Worries about certain types of foods.

- Feeling sluggish and lethargic after overeating.

- Dealing with negative feelings after overeating.

- Having some withdrawal symptoms including agitation or anxiety when cutting down or stopping to eat certain foods

- Difficulty in functioning effectively with daily routines, job / School, social and family activities.

Industrial and commercially prepared foods have been proven by many studies to be addictive:

- Sugar stimulates the brain's reward centers through the neurotransmitter dopamine exactly like other addictive substances.

- PET imaging shows that high-sugar and high-fat foods work just like heroin, opium and morphine in the brain.

- The numbers of dopamine receptors are reduced in both obese individuals and drug addicts, according to results from PET brain imaging, thus, they have to crave things to boost dopamine.

- Research has shown that sugary and fatty foods stimulate the release of body's own opioids in the brain.

- Drugs (medications) used to block the brain's receptors for heroin and morphine can also reduce the cravings for consumption of high-sugar and high-fat foods.

- People can become tolerant to sugar, and need more and more for satisfaction, similar to drugs of abuse and alcohol.

- Obese people continue to eat large amounts of unhealthy foods despite serious social and personal negative consequences, just like drug addicts and alcoholics.

- After the initial period of enjoyment of certain foods, the eaters no longer consume the foods to get ' high ', but to feel normal, just like the illegal drugs.

- People addicted to sugar can experience withdrawal when suddenly cut off from it, just like drug addicts and alcoholics detoxifying.

For normal-weight people, an empty stomach triggers the brain to tell the body to get some food; when the stomach is full, it gets happy and that is the end of that for about 5 hours or more. Some obese people, however, find themselves eating again only an hour or so after a meal. Therefore, food cravings may be particularly relevant to people with obesity. Studies have suggested that the brains of obese people have poor appetite control, so they are more intensely hungry than naturally thin people. The brains of obese people tend to respond more strongly to food cues, even in the absence of hunger.

In a study of 15 lean women and 15 obese women with functional MRI scans before and after a meal, researchers found that lean women are very aware of food when they are hungry, but after they eat, they can think about other things. Obese women are very aware of food all the time.

Researchers from the University of Granada in Spain and Monash University in Australia compared the difference in functional connectivity between the reward centers of the brain and obese people. They found that food cravings activate different networks and that the desire for food may actually be hardwired into the brains of overweight and obese people.

Most of us cannot deny that obesity has become a major health problem in the U.S., and most of the efforts of treatment have remained relatively unsuccessful. By some estimates, up to 80% of people who successfully lost weight gradually regained it to end up as heavy or even heavier than they were before they went on a diet.

Recent scientific studies are beginning to understand the brain-related mechanisms associated with overeating and obesity similar to chemical dependency, and are trying to develop an approach in the same manner as alcohol or drug addiction. The Food and Drug Administration of the U.S. Government has recently approved a new, pharmaceutical combination of naltrexone and bupropion for the treatment of obesity, after several large studies showing their anti-craving effect for obese patients.

Before resorting to prescription medications to help you with your cravings and overweight problems, there are a few things you can do to help hold your cravings in check:

    Get sufficient sleep every night. In a University of Chicago study, a few sleepless nights were enough to reduce the levels of the hormone leptin, which signals satiety, by 18% and boost the levels of ghrelin, the appetite trigger, by a whopping 30%. These two changes alone can cause your appetite to kick into overdrive and cravings for starchy foods like cookies and bread by 45%.

- Eliminate sensory cues. We need to know that smell, sights and sounds all act as powerful triggers. Try to stay away from the kitchen, which may be full of snacks, after dinners. Read a book or do a cross-word puzzle in the basement, or listen to some of your favorite music to relax before bedtime, or find some interesting articles in the magazines. Do not put your favorite treats on the kitchen counter.

- Try not to buy and keep those tempting foods at home because they are too easy and convenient and difficult to stop. Instead, go out for your ice cream or your piece of pizza, as long as you have learnt portion control. Having a little bit of what you crave is a good way to break the craving because feeling deprived of a favorite food often backfires and you can end up eating too much. You may find that just a little taste will satisfy your craving!

  According to research from the University of Toronto, restrained eaters are very likely to experience cravings and to overeat the ' forbidden ' food when given a chance. In a study published in the journal Appetite, women who were asked to cut carbs for three days reported stronger food cravings and ate 44% more calories from carb-rich foods on day 4. It is better to enjoy a little bit of your favorite treats with portion control so that you don't feel deprived and sorry for yourself.

- The brain-gut connection. The bacteria found in your gut, the intestinal tract, may be affecting both your cravings and mood, and may even push you toward obesity, according to a new analysis published in the journal BioEssays. Based on the scientific studies from the University of California, San

Francisco, Arizona State University, and University of New Mexico, the microbes living in your digestive tract can cause you to crave particular nutrients they need to grow on.

Some bacterial species thrive on fat, and other sugar, for example. They compete with each other for food and try to retain a niche within their ecosystem (your intestinal tract). Science has confirmed that the gut is linked to the immune system, the nervous system and the endocrine system. The signals released by these bacteria can influence your physiologic and behavioral responses.

Your diets, however, have a significant impact on the microbial population in your gut. This microbiome is quick and adaptable to changes. Having a healthy balance of these gut bacteria may allow you to lead a healthy life and lower your risk of obesity.

- Take a walk. A University of Exeter study found that walking briskly for 15 minutes reduced cravings for chocolate – the most commonly reported food craving – during the walk and for at least 15 minute afterward. Researchers reported that exercise could alter brain chemicals that help regulate cravings.

- Play a game on your smart phone as little as three minutes could get your mind off food. In a study in Addictive Behaviors, participants reported when they had cravings for food, alcohol and more, their craving levels dropped by about 20% after playing the game, which seemed to occupy the mental process and displaced the cravings.

- Relaxation. Stresses flood your body with the hormone cortisol, triggering the urge to eat food high in fat and sugar. Studies have shown that meditation and yoga can decrease stress and make it easier to resist binge eating and cravings. Do not let emotional eating undermine your diet.

Ĭ   Make a fist. For some reasons, tightening your muscles can give your will power a lift. In a Journal of Consumer Research study, participants who clenched their fists, tightened their biceps or stretch their fingers while making food choices picked healthier foods than those who did not. The researchers suggested that firming up your muscles while trying to exert self-control could strengthen your resolve.

Why do so many people regain weight after they have worked so hard to lose it? This sad and discouraging phenomenon has puzzled dieters and obesity researchers for many years. The newest research posits that it is your ' appetite ' that can sabotage your weight loss.

People who have lost weight tend to get really hungry with a surge in appetite, more than the decrease in metabolism people have after weight loss. The surge in appetite drives the regain of body weight because the effect of the appetite surge is three times stronger than the slowing metabolism, according to obesity research.

Experts have been trying to understand why it is so difficult to maintain weight loss. Many have agreed that one of the most important parts of the equation is food intake after weight loss. According to many studies, people are notoriously bad at keeping track of how much they eat. One study found that people trying to lose weight only thought they were eating almost half as much as they actually were.

Let us look at the side of food intake in this equation; personally, I think food intake is the most crucial part of the equation, others including but limited to exercise, mental health, genetics, environments and lifestyles. After all, you are what you eat! The following list of foods will keep you full and help fight those sugar and insulin spikes and crashes that can make it difficult to control your cravings and stick to your diet.

- Black beans. Their high protein and soluble fiber contents make them a great fighter for anyone trying to fend off cravings. They will keep your full and your blood sugar levels stable, but not bloated.

- Chickpeas. These legumes help keep your cravings from getting out of hand in two ways. First, their high protein content keeps you full for longer than the average carb-rich food. Second, they have been known to reduce blood sugar levels, according to a study in the Archives of Internal Medicine, meaning you are less hungry and less likely to go seeking a quick carb-heavy fix.

- Pineapples. They are low on the scale of glycemic index, meaning it will not raise your blood sugar as rapidly as other fruits and definitely will not cause the crash you will get from sweet foods that contained refined sugar.

- Salmon. It is carb-free and full of omega-3 fatty acids. The fish is also rich in protein, keeping your sugar from going crazy and avoiding cravings.

- Quinoa. These little things are full of protein and fiber, ideal for weight loss. Research published in the Journal of Food Science and Technology indicates that quinoa has powerful. Positive effect on eating behaviors.

- Blueberries. They are sweet but have a low glycemic index, making them a great addition to any diet where blood sugar spikes are a concern. A serving of blueberries has nearly 4 grams of fiber, which will keep you full long enough to quell those food cravings. Research published in the

British Medical Journal also indicate that their antioxidants/ flavonoids may help you maintain healthy weight.

- Probiotic yogurt. Its healthy protein and beneficial bacteria help you feeling full and keep you blood sugar from spiking, promoting healthy weight.

- Apples. An apple a day, not only keeps the doctor away, it also keeps those cravings away. Apples have been shown to have a satiating effect and reduce the incidence of overeating, while providing plenty of fiber to keep you feeling full.

- Black coffee. Moderation consumption of black coffee has many health benefits. It has been shown to reduce blood sugar levels and may even keep you from becoming diabetic later in life. It helps to keep you energized and minimize food cravings.

- Oatmeal. A wonderful member of the whole grain family. Oatmeal can help you lose weight, curb your cravings and improve your cardiovascular health. A study published in the American Journal of Clinical Nutrition found that whole grains help reduce risk of blood sugar-related conditions like diabetes.

- Grapefruit. A must and a superfood for weight-loss enthusiasts. It can curb your cravings, facilitate your weight loss efforts and lower your blood sugar at the same time, according to research published in the Journal of Medicinal Food.

- Lemons. This aromatic fruit can reduce blood sugar and insulin resistance, helping you lose weight with its polyphenols, according to many studies.

- Green tea. Its fat-burning effects have been well-documented. In addition to an energy burst from caffeine, green teas also provides polysaccharides and catechins, both of which can fire up your metabolism while boosting your body's ability to process sugar and keeping your blood sugar levels stable over a prolonged period of time. So, when you have a craving, go for a cup of green tea instead.

- Cinnamon. This spice is a mighty soldier against cravings. A study published in Diabetes Care found that cinnamon significantly lowered blood sugar levels of diabetic subjects as well as reducing bad cholesterol and other risk factors for heart disease. It is also a rich source of antioxidants and should be part of your diet.

- Kiwi. It has a very low glycemic index, and is ideal to fight cravings in your weight loss endeavor.

- Artichokes. Their leaves are the healthiest sources of fiber, helping to keep you full while lowering the blood sugar. A study published in the Journal of Medicinal Food found that consumption of artichokes has a profound antidiabetic effect, stabilizing blood sugar while curbing cravings.

- Pomegranate. Foods like pomegranate that take a while to eat can help your blood sugar maintain an even keel while giving your brain enough time to realize that your stomach is full. This fruit is a powerful weapon against sugar spikes and is listed as one of the best fruits for a flat belly.

- Ginger. It is rich in antioxidants, and has powerful anti-inflammatory effects. More and more scientific evidence has shown that inflammation is a precursor of obesity; ginger can do more than just settling your stomach, it can also regulate your blood sugar to minimize your cravings and decrease overeating.

- Kale. This dark leafy green has many health benefits; it also has anti-diabetic and anti-inflammatory effects, stabilizing the blood sugar and promoting healthy weight by diminishing your cravings.

- Tomatoes. A natural fat fighter due to the high content of vitamin C, 9-oxo-ODA and riboflavin. Research has shown that low energy-density foods like tomatoes influence eaters to eat less, promoting the feeling of satisfaction.

- Almonds. Lots of health benefits with little money. They keep you feeling full, protect your heart, lower your blood pressure, reduce your cholesterol and can help stave off your cravings thanks to their high levels of protein, fiber and heart-healthy fat. This is the snack you should be carrying around with you, especially when you have cravings.

- Avocados. They are considered one of the best fruits for weight loss and a flat belly. With their high content of heart-healthy fat, protein and fiber, you will fell fuller for longer. A study published in Nutrition Journal found that people who ate avocado with their meal reported greater satiety and had more stable blood sugar levels than those who went without avocados.

- Eggs. Inexpensive source of protein with many other health benefits, eggs will keep you from feeling hungry without promoting sugar and insulin spikes. Dieters should include this low-carb food on their list.

- Peanuts. Try to go for the unsalted or low-salt ones. According to studies published in the Journal of the American College of Nutrition, consumption of peanuts can help reduce sugar and insulin spikes, leading to less cravings and overall food intake.

- Lentils. These small things are rich in soluble fiber, about 16grams per cup. It can keep your blood sugar from spiking and avoid cravings. Lentils are a must-have for any long-term weight loss program.

- Brown rice. Its complex carbohydrate coupled with a fiber-rich protein will keep you full and satiated longer than its white counterparts. Try to stay away from white rice if you can.

- Sweet potatoes. They are naturally sweet but able to keep your blood sugar levels in check and your carvings to a minimum. Its high content of beta-carotene has many health benefits.

- Pecans. They are a great source of antioxidants, protein and fiber, helping to stop spikes of your blood sugar. Their plant sterols can lower cholesterol as an added bonus, promoting healthy weight and heart.

- Curry. A healthy spice popular in the Eastern diets. It has sugar-stabilizing effect like cinnamon and cloves, good for minimizing cravings and weight loss.

- Cashews. Crunchy and tasty nuts with lots of protein and heart-healthy fat to keep your blood sugar from rising to craving-provoking levels.

- Wheat germs. They are high-fiber complex carbohydrates, very effective in keeping blood sugar levels stable to prevent cravings.

⏳ Cherries. Their high levels of fat-fighting resveratrol may help keep your cravings to a minimum. They contain a compound, called anthocyanin, which can improve the efficacy of your body's insulin while keeping your blood levels under control. Their antioxidants are very anti-inflammatory, promoting healthy weight against obesity.

Some of you may be wondering why your scale is not going down even though you consider yourself diligent about your eating habits – eating mostly fruits and vegetables with some lean meats. You are active, without unhealthy lifestyles and able to handle your cravings, but you are still not losing weight.

Have you thought about your favorite condiments which can be the precursors to weight gain, working against your weight loss efforts? Actually, many of the common condiments out there can be to blame; unfortunately, most people do not seem to know enough about them except for the sugar and salt packets and use them innocently over time. To tell you the truth, many of the common condiments are a recipe for weight gain. Here is a list of some common ones you should be aware of besides sugar and salt:

⏳ Ketchup. It comes from one of the two most-consumed vegetables in the United States, tomatoes. Ketchup consumption is out of control, and this ketchup is far from the nutritional equivalent of enjoying a healthy salad with fresh tomatoes.

   Most ketchup is heavily sweetened with obesity-promoting added sugar and high fructose corn syrup.

⏳ Mayonnaise. It is loaded with saturated fat and preservatives, and its consumption will definitely lead to packing on the pounds.

- Barbecue sauce. It is packed with sugar, plus other salty ingredients like soy sauce.

- Mexican sauce. It is prepared with chocolate, added sugar, white bread and even lard.

- Ranch dressing. It contains dairy and high-salt ingredients, promoting bloating. Some are mixed with sour cream and mayonnaise, densely caloric.

- Tomato sauce. It sounds like a healthy condiment, but much of what you can buy in the store is far from healthy. Most of the popular brands are packed with sugar or high fructose corn syrup, as well as unhealthy amounts of salt, artificial color and preservatives. All of these ingredients will add up to a lot of pounds over time.

- Peanut sauce. Peanuts are healthy legumes in their natural form, but when it is processed with lots of added sugar and other additives, it is a different story. Stay away if you are serious about losing weight.

- French dressing. Another seemingly healthy topping for your salad, in reality, it is a combination of ketchup, sugar, vinegar and fattening oil.

- Pancake syrup. This sweet liquid is made from high fructose corn syrup, artificial coloring and oil, nothing like the real maple syrup from the sap of the tree.

- Black bean sauce. The black beans in the name actually refer to fermented soybeans, which can cause a variety of health problems. When you add in sugar and omega-6 fats, you have got trouble including obesity.

- Blue cheese dressing. Many brands are loaded with salt, artificial colors, and toxic preservatives like sodium benzoate and phosphoric acid. It is high in calories and low in nutritional value. It is not something to pour over your fresh salad because it will offset all of the health benefits of the fresh vegetables plus more.

- Italian dressing. Another seemingly benign item for your healthy salad. It is a mixture of sugar, high fructose corn syrup with vegetable oil and spices.

- Teriyaki sauce. A very popular sauce for quite a few entrée, but it is mainly a mixture of sugar, rice wine, soy sauce and garlic. It is a recipe for blood sugar spike, hunger and cravings, making it very difficult for the dieters.

- Jelly. At least 60% of sugar across the board, according to the Department of Agriculture of the U.S., plus other unhealthy additives.

- Sour cream. This popular condiment is highly calorific with a lot of salt and other additives.

- Cocktail sauce. A companion of shrimp, which is on the list of the World's Healthiest Seafood. The cocktail sauce, in actuality, makes very bad companion for the shrimp, when it is prepared and combined with sugar-laden ketchup, salty hot sauce, and horseradish.. By the way, the horseradish in cocktail sauce may have a goitrogenic effect; people with thyroid problems must be extra careful using this sauce.

- Wasabi sauce. It is prepared with mostly horseradish in most brands, and if you have a diagnosis of thyroid problem, it is best to avoid it.

- Honey mustard. This popular liquid condiment is made with high fructose corn syrup, one of the major culprits for obesity.

- Relish. Just about everybody adds it onto their hot dogs and other foods. Though low in calorie, it is loaded with sugar and salt, not good for anyone who is trying to lose weight.

- Soy sauce. Soy may be a probiotic powerhouse, but when you add a lot of salt and other things to it, it is ruined adverse impact on health.

- Hoisin sauce. A popular condiment for Chinese foods, but it is loaded with sugar and sodium, and will add back the pounds you might have lost.

- Plum sauce. Another common liquid condiment, popular in Chinese restaurants. It is essentially sugar gravy along with corn starch and dangerous omega-6 oil.

- Steak sauce. Most of the brands are loaded with sugar and/or high fructose corn syrup. It is acceptable and understandable to enjoy a piece of lean, grass-fed steak occasionally, but it is better to do it with little amount of the sauce. Again, this is portion control. There is a saying: there is no bad food, there is only bad portion.

- Mint jelly. When you are loading up your lamb chops with mint jelly, you might as well be pouring pancake syrup all over them. The mint jelly does have some healthy mint in it, the rest of its recipe is artificial coloring, lots of added sugar and vinegar. So, be mindful and go easy with it.

CHAPTER TEN

Obesity and poverty

Is obesity a disease of the poor in the U.S.? Is poverty linked to obesity? Do obesity and poverty always go together?

These are difficult questions to answer sometimes; and these questions, to some people, may have some implications of political correctness. Before we get into the crux of the matter, let us look at some interesting findings concerning the world's five fattest and five thinnest countries based on BMI criteria. Public health researchers define obesity and overweight more generally in terms of BMI, standing for basal metabolic index. A person's BMI is his or her weight in kilograms divided by the square of his or her height in meters. A BMI of 25 or more is considered overweight; 30 or more is considered obese.

Tonga

This Polynesian state wins the battle of the bulge; in actuality, the people of Tonga have a lot to lose, looking at it from health standpoint. About 86.1 percent of its population are overweight or obese. It is no wonder their type-2 diabetes rate sits sadly around 40 percent.

Traditionally, this island state's diet consisted of fish, root vegetables and coconuts, but in the middle of the twentieth century, things began to change. Processed meats, sugary drinks and other commercialized food products started to arrive in the middle of the twentieth century. Along with the lack of education regarding healthy foods up until recent decades, obesity problem has been ballooning to become a nation with the highest percentage of fat people.

American Samoa

The World Health Organization lists American Samoa's overweight and obesity rate at 84%, but some health officials claim that it could be as high as 90%. The situation is really pitiful and dangerous; it is so out of hand that the airline, Samoa Air, has actually made the local people stand on the scales with their luggage so they can pay according to their weight.

The primary cause of this is the cost of food, especially the healthy food such as quality meat and fresh produce which are usually imported. The cheap alternative is fast food, which is the case in most of the world. The government of American Samoa is trying to get their people in shape through public service announcements and healthy eating education in school in order to save the future generations, but they have a long way to go.

Kiribati

The people of this island republic in the Central Pacific have been replacing their food with packaged and processed high-calorie foods in the past two decades, causing the weight of the people to soar. It is made worse with their notoriously sedentary lifestyles, leading the nation to the current overweight/obesity rate of 79.1%.

Kuwait

A few decades ago, this mid-eastern nation was a farming country, whose residents often performed manual labor, worked on farms, and ate fresh local food. However, the discovery of Kuwait's huge crude oil reserves has made it quite prosperous, and the change means the people are working less and having more money to spend, almost like a windfall.

Moreover, fast food chains came and established themselves with the arrival of the U.S. troops during the first Gulf War. Restaurants such as McDonald's and Pizza Hut are so popular, and have become part of an unhealthy lifestyle unfortunately. Leading the nation to the current overweight/obesity rate of 78.1%

Qatar

This small nation in the Middle East has been ranked in the top of the fattest nations in the world for quite a few years, currently with 77.1% of the population listed as overweight and obese. The cause for this alarming phenomenon is obvious, thanks to its enormous crude oil reserves.

For a country that is smaller than Connecticut but has a million more people, work is difficult to find, and most of the people lead sedentary lifestyles. More and more people in Qatar are relying on automobiles for transportation, and eating most of the meals at the popular fast food chains. With its trends continuing without concerted efforts to change course, Qatar will stay at the top of the obesity list for a long time.

North Korea

According to available data, most of the people in this country are literally starving, earning an average of less than $30 per month. North Korean food is relatively healthy; the diet generally includes rice, noodles, corn porridge, kimchi, soybean sausages and bulgogi. With the ongoing famine and political unrest, there is just not enough food to go around, leading North Korea to be the thinnest nation on earth with a shockingly low 4.4% overweight/obesity rate.

East Timor

This Southeast Asian country, like their neighbors, has a diet that mostly features local pork, fish, basil, legumes, corn, rice root vegetables and tropical fruit. Unfortunately, these healthy food items are scarce, and the situations are made worse with much political unrest and turmoil, leading to widespread malnourishment in rural areas. Thus, the overweight/obesity rate of East Timor has remained extremely low at 4.9%.

Ethiopia

This African nation is unfortunately known for hunger, malnourishment, poor sanitary conditions, and high mortality rates in children. Complicated with political unrest, there simply is not enough food to go around, keeping the overweight/obesity rate low at 6.1%. For the residents lucky enough to have enough to eat, the food they consume is rather healthy, thanks to the large amount of agriculture – which makes up at least 40% of the GDP.

The conditions are improving slowly, especially in the cities where health statistics are better across the board.

Vietnam

In general, the Vietnamese diet is low in fat and sugar, and is loaded with vitamins, minerals and antioxidants. This is positive and encouraging, giving Vietnam a 13.1 percent overweight/obesity rate, despite the fact that it is not a wealthy nation in Southeast Asia with inadequate government funding of health care and shortages of doctors, nurses, hospitals and clinics, especially in the rural areas.

However, the conditions seem to be improving, with the country's life expectancy rate increased to a healthy 76 years for women and 72 for men recently.

Madagascar

This island republic in the Indian Ocean off the southeastern coast of Africa has a population of about 14 million people. This island nation is, oftentimes, adversely affected by natural disasters like floods, cyclones and drought. Almost 36% of the rural population suffers from food insecurity, and about two million children are stunted because of chronic malnutrition. Its overweight/obesity rate is only a little over 11%. Locals are seriously underweight from birth, making it fifth in the world in regard to underweight children.

Health services have shown some improvement in the last 20 years, in particular, immunizations, along with living conditions and food supplies, slowly raising the life expectancy rate.

Now we have a glimpse of some of the weight problems other nations are facing outside the U.S. Globally speaking, high-income countries seem to have greater rates of obesity than low-income countries. Countries that develop wealth and economic growth also develop obesity, and prime examples include China and India where obesity rates have increased by several folds.

Ironically, in America, obesity seems to be more prevalent in impoverished areas than communities with higher income. The U.S. is one of the wealthiest nations in the world; but one third of the population is obese and another third is overweight. In the U.S., how is poverty linked to obesity? In other words, why is obesity so common among the poor?

Obesity varies considerably depending on gender, race, ethnicity and socioeconomic factors. Among women, obesity is most prevalent at lower income levels: 42% of women living in households with income below 130% of the poverty are obese. In the U.S., poverty thresholds are set every year by the Census Bureau, and vary by family size and composition. According to the most recent government report, 2011-12, it was found that obesity was significantly more common among black women than black men, there was far less obesity among Asian Americans than other racial/ethnic groups.

Obesity in early childhood raises the risks of obesity in teenage years and later in life; parents are very influential and have the power to address and change the issue. Children from the wealthiest 20% of families have the lowest prevalence of obesity in kindergarten compared with those from all other socioeconomic groups, according to a study recently published in the New England Journal of Medicine. The poorer a child is, the more likely he or she is to be overweight at a very young age; and the trend will get worse as they proceed to adolescence.

According to a paper recently released in the Proceedings of the National Academy of Sciences, there is a socioeconomic health gap among children, and the gap is widening. It is undeniable that obesity is a major health concern, or public health issue for poor children. According to research published in Harvard Business Review, between 2003 and 2010, obesity rate among teens whose parents have no more than a high-school education rose from about 20% to 25%. Over the same period, obesity rates among teenagers whose parents had a 4-year college degree or more declined from 14% to about 7%.

There is no question that the rates of obesity and type-2 diabetes in the U.S. follow a socioeconomic gradient, such that the burden of disease falls disproportionately on people with limited resources, racial/ethnic minorities (except for the Asian Americans) and the poor.

Among women, higher obesity rates tend to be associated with low income and low education levels, although obesity rates have continued to increase for men and women and at all educational levels, the highest rates occur among the most disadvantaged groups.

Personal and parental responsibilities have a role in addressing the childhood obesity crisis, the roots of the problem extend much farther and deeper. Relying only on personal and parental responsibilities and individual decision without considering other factors will change nothing.

Let us look at some of the other factors that adversely impact obesity, especially childhood obesity, among the low-income people:

- People who live in impoverished regions have poor access to fresh food in general. These poor areas are sometimes called ' food desert ', and the residents are often hungry and unable to find affordable healthy foods. This phenomenon is known as food insecurity, meaning poor access to food including healthy ones by low-income households.

- Studies have shown that people living in poor areas are less active with sedentary lifestyle, which, we know, is prone to obesity. The confined, sedentary lifestyle is due, in part, to increased violence and crime rates in impoverished regions, thereby preventing parents and children from being active outdoors or venturing out of their homes. Another factor is the high unemployment rates among the poor folks without or with minimum goal-oriented activities and productive routines like a job.

- Lack of park with facilities and setup for physical activity, sports and exercise. At least, these things are less available to people living in the poor areas; and the poor residents may be less able to afford gym membership, sports clothing and/or exercise equipment. Even if the facilities are available, parents themselves and their children are concerned about their safety.

- The low cost of energy-dense foods promotes consumption in the poor areas; and the selection of these energy-dense foods by the food-insecure and low-income households may represent a deliberate strategy to save money. People trying to limit food costs will first choose less expensive but more energy-dense foods to maintain dietary energy.

Many studies have shown that energy-dense foods have been associated with decreased satiation and satiety, overconsumption of fats and sweets, and overall higher energy intakes. Usually, energy-dense foods are more palatable, providing more sensory enjoyment and more pleasure than do foods that are not. Typically, less expensive, energy-dense foods have lower nutritional quality and, with over-consumption, have been linked to obesity.

Clinical studies have found that the most likely targets of food cravings are those foods contain fat, sugar or both. Human taste preference for sugar and fat are either innate or acquired very early in life. Children preferred the more energy-dense foods and gave higher ratings to chocolate cookies and chips than to vegetables and fruit. Food preference, according to many scientific studies, can be shaped by repeated exposures and influenced by parents through their own preferences.

In a recent study, mothers indicated that their children liked energy-dense foods such as pizza, chocolate chip cookies and sweetened breakfast cereals, whereas low energy-dense foods like tomatoes, cucumbers, broccoli and cabbage were disliked by children and their mothers.

Ⓧ Aggressive food advertising and marketing on TV and social media have been cited as a factor contributing to a higher energy and fat intake. In 1997, food manufacturers, food retailers and food service companies reportedly spent eleven billion dollars on advertising, much of it on foods with added sugars and fat. With more competition nowadays for market share, the force of advertising and marketing has become stronger and pervasive, making it hard to ignore. These frequent sensory bombardments have a profound effect on anyone, especially the impressionable children. One research shows that low-income youths and adults are exposed to disproportionately more marketing and advertising that encourage the consumption of unhealthy foods.

Ⓧ Fast food restaurants seem to be very visible and accessible in many low-income communities. These eateries typically serve many energy-dense, nutrient-poor processed foods at relatively low prices. They also make larger portion sizes more tempting for your dollar. Studies have demonstrated that consumption of fast food often lead to weight gain. Research shows that more and more people are eating their meals away from home. Cooking and mindfully preparing your meals at home is surely the best way to keep overweight and obesity at bay.

⚰ Feast or famine situation is often found in low-income households which are trying to stretch food budgets. They, including children, may overeat when food is available, especially after skipping a meal. Research shows that parental obesity is a strong predictor of childhood obesity.

⚰ The increased levels of stress in impoverished neighborhood tend to promote poor eating habits and lead to poor mental health such as depression. This sad combination is a certain, speedy path to obesity, as shown in many research studies which have linked poor mental health and stress to obesity in children and adults. A number of other studies have also found association between maternal stress or depression and childhood obesity. Stress and poor mental health may lead to weight gain and obesity through stress-induced hormonal and metabolic changes as well as unhealthy eating habits and physical inactivity.

⚰ Transportation logistics are not favorable for people living in the poor areas. Even though walking is one of the healthiest physical activities to help maintaining healthy weight, it is probably not a safe option for them due to various reasons such as increased violence and crime. Many may not have the fund to own their own automobiles, and paying for taxi rides can be very costly. Public transportation may be available but time-consuming and encumbered by bad weather sometimes. So, children from low-income households are less likely to participate in organized sports.

⚰ Low-income neighborhoods, in general, lack full-service grocery stores and farmers markets, where residents and purchase high-quality fruits, vegetables, wholegrains and low-fat dairy products. The situation is made worse when they do not have reliable means of transportation. They are thus limited to the small neighborhood convenience and corner stores, often with higher prices and less choices. Their food purchase and choices are further constrained by limits on how much they can carry when walking or using public transportation. According to USDA, vehicle availability is perhaps the most important determinant of whether or not a family can access affordable and nutritious foods.

☉ Healthy foods including organic items are generally more expensive, whereas refined grains, added sugar and fats are generally inexpensive, palatable and readily available in low-income neighborhoods. These less expensive energy-dense foods typically have less nutritional value and are unhealthy and fattening.

☉ Despite many positive changes in the healthcare industry, many low-income people still have limited access to health care, in particular, preventive medical care, resulting in lack of or insufficient screening, as well as lack of diagnosis and treatment of emerging chronic health problems like obesity. Referrals from these neighborhood clinics to medical specialists may require distant travel and can be time-consuming, and patients from poor neighborhoods may not be motivated to overcome different barriers.

The link between obesity, especially childhood obesity, and poverty may be too costly to ignore because obesity-related chronic diseases already account for about 70% of the health care costs, perhaps more. These chronic diseases include diabetes, high blood pressure, hyperlipidemia, sleep disorders, arthritis, asthma, premature aging, some types of cancer, and cardiovascular disease.

Obesity is a serious problem, and has become an epidemic requiring aggressive combat strategies from all fronts. Obesity soared in the U.S. during 1980s and 1990s, doubling among adults and tripling among children. The obesity epidemic appears to have hit a plateau, according to the latest federal data. The proportion of adult Americans who are obese held steady at 35% and there is some evidence that the overall obesity rate had leveled off since 2004, probably due to the attention the problem has been getting. Whatever it is, the plateau is welcome news, I hope it will eventually trend down as the beginning of a positive movement.

With one-third of American adults and almost 17% of children and adolescents are still obese (more than 78 million adults and more than 12.7 million children and adolescents), our country is still facing a daunting task and a wave of medical problems related to obesity.

Our country is resourceful, resilient and compassionate; we just need to cooperate and work together for the common good, which is the healthy children, our future. This problem of obesity does not require advanced technologies for diagnosis and treatments. A triangular approach with the government leading at the top, with the families and the private sectors on both sides supporting healthy governmental initiatives. It takes a village to raise a healthy child!

Is obesity the government's business? In my view, it is a resounding ' yes '. Obesity is a public health issue and the problem has reached an epidemic proportion. It is in our government's interest to develop a well-rounded, proactive and aggressive strategy to combat the problem. Some people have argued and are still arguing against governmental intrusion into our personal habits and freedom of choice.

This is nothing new, and our government has tried to encourage all of us to pursue a healthy and fit nation. Dr. David Satcher, who served as the 16th Surgeon General of the U.S. from 1988 to 2001, published America's first " Call to Action to Prevent and Decrease Overweight and Obesity ".

It is very encouraging and laudable that the federal government has made prevention and treatment of obesity a major part of its campaign in 2010 to improve the health of America by launching a series of initiatives that are likely to have a long-term impact on stemming the tide of obesity in the U.S. On February 09, 2010, the first lady Michelle Obama unveiled her Let's Move campaign to combat childhood obesity.

The first lady's Let's Move campaign represents a major turning point in the nation's fight against obesity, particularly, childhood obesity. President Obama and the first lady have made healthier living a national priority through the Let's Move campaign, which enjoys broad bipartisan support.

The Let's Move campaign is committed to ending ' food deserts ' (i.e. communities without full-service supermarkets and farmers markets) within seven years, while promoting healthier foods in schools, thus addressing two major challenges in healthier living.

The recent enactment of health care reform also will play an important role in combating obesity. For one provision, the legislation provides $500 million for prevention and wellness grants in 2010, an amount to increase to $15 billion during the next ten years. Another provision of the legislation will require any restaurant with 20 or more locations to include calorie counts on individual menus, menu boards and drive through menus. The provision, which took effect in 2011, also will apply to foods sold in vending machines. The FDA is responsible for enforcing the requirements.

The menu labeling requirements have a big impact on the choices of food consumers make and even on the formulation of food. The first goal of menu labeling is public information for the consumers because most calories nowadays are consumed outside of the homes. Hopefully, with menu labeling, consumers are more likely to change their food choices, prompting restaurants to alter their food formulations to make them healthier.

Healthier food and snacks, and safe and proper physical activity should be mandated of all child care facilities across the board, since more than 12 million children regularly spend time at child care centers outside the homes. However, not all states use licensing regulations to ensure that the children are provided healthier food and snacks with supervised activities.

Federal and local taxation policies on certain consumer products can be a powerful tool to fight against obesity. Beverages with added sugar are a prime candidate for taxation. As we know, sugary beverages have little or no nutritional value, and consumption of them is associated with weight gain and obesity and other related health problems. Taxes on sugary drinks have been gaining interest and some support across nation. In fact, all sugary beverages should be banned from elementary and secondary schools, both private and public; some of the schools have already done so for the health of the students.

Our country is founded on democracy with a strong love and sentiment for freedom, especially the first amendment. The U.S. government has taken some steps to address the issue of advertising and marketing of junk foods with recommendations for nutritional quality standards for food marketed to children 12 and younger.

Healthier lunches and breakfasts should be mandated and enforced at all public schools at elementary and secondary levels. Initial reactions from the parents and students may not be satisfactory or pleasant because this is cultural and it takes time and repeated exposures to change. Therefore, nutritional education is critical and should be required for the children and adolescents so they will understand and appreciate what they eat.

Some people do not like the financial support given to the farmers by the federal government in the form of agricultural subsidies to grow or raise certain products including corn, soybeans, wheat, rice, sorghum. dairy and livestock. In contrast, subsidies for legumes, fruit and vegetables are very minimal, and almost non-existent. Agricultural subsidies are grossly skewed, according to government data, creating a diet excessively high in factory-farmed meats, grains and sugars with very little fresh fruits and vegetables or healthy fats from nuts and seeds. Some opponents of agricultural subsidies consider the subsidies roots of our society's health problems with obesity because Americans get more than half of their daily calories from those seven farm foods that are subsidized by the U.S. government. A recent study suggests that those subsidies may be contributing to the obesity epidemic.

They claimed that by subsidizing the farming of corn and soy, our government is actually supporting a diet that consists of these grains in their processed form, namely high fructose corn syrup, soybean oil and grain-fed cattle – all of which are known contributors to obesity and chronic diseases. The issue of agricultural subsidies is a complex one, with political overtone and global trade involvements. This ideological issue is not easy to understand and resolve unfortunately. As consumers, we must be more knowledgeable, proactive and discerning.

With the leadership of our governments, federal, state and local, park areas should be made gun-free zones, like the schools, especially in impoverished communities, so that parents are not afraid to accompany their children to play and run at the parks, and adolescents can play sports at the park.

Nutrition classes should be a requirement at both public elementary and secondary schools; healthy lifestyle and eating habits should be taught early in life in order to change the undesirable culture of eating mindlessly.

Parents of the children should make the healthy food choices for their impressionable children. Due to lower educational levels of parents in low-income neighborhoods, public education is crucial for the parents in the communities with government funding and faith-based charities. We know parents have considerable influence on the children and if they can be exemplary, it will be a good beginning for the children. If the parents are obese, it is hard for the children to keep healthy weight.

Basic classes of food economics should be given to parents so that they can become better consumers, getting the best value out of their food budget. Not all healthy foods are expensive, and they can learn to get the most nutrition from foods inexpensively.

There should be home visiting nurses to observe the kitchen and teach parents in food preparations, and the use of healthy condiments. Many condiments used at home are fattening and most consumers are not aware of it. Education regarding use of sugar, salt and cooking oils should be done and emphasized; they are major culprits for weight gain.

Home education should include avoidance or cut-down of fried and grilled foods, and increased consumption of fruit and vegetables. The approach and instruction should be simple and basic, and easy to understand and follow. During home visits, signs and symptoms of mental health should be observed, and referrals to mental health professionals made when necessary. Poor mental health and poverty will often lead to obesity.

Local healthcare providers should encourage and support young mothers to breast feed their babies. Most mothers started out breast-feeding, by the end of six months, only 13% or less of babies are exclusively breast-fed. Family, healthcare providers, employers, and community should support breast-feeding because it is the best food for the developing babies. And the intimate bonding between the mother and the baby has far-reaching benefits.

Local healthcare providers should provide diet education, preventive care and screening for patients who have high risk for obesity. Keeping excess weight off and maintaining healthy weight is not easy, and there are many disappointing and unsuccessful stories. You just need to keep trying, one pound at a time. People wanting and trying to lose weight, especially those living in impoverished areas, need encouragement, respect, education, mutual understanding, family support, and positive social interactions, in addition to various government programs.

CHAPTER ELEVEN

Obesity and Fatty Liver

Belly fat or visceral fat correlates well with fatty liver disease, especially in middle-aged adults, according to Research Center for Non-Alcoholic Fatty Liver Disease (NAFLD) at the University of California at San Diego. High levels of triglycerides or LDL cholesterol signal there is too much fat in your liver. People who are overweight or obese are at an increased risk of NAFLD. When BMI goes up, the prevalence of NAFLD also goes up.

The normal amount of body fat expressed as a percentage of body weight is between 25% and 30% in women and 18% and 23% in men. This is just another way of defining obesity.

The liver is a vital glandular organ, located in the right upper quadrant of the abdomen below the diaphragm. It has multiple functions, including detoxification of various metabolites, protein synthesis, and the production of different biochemical compounds necessary for digestion. One of those is bile, which is an alkaline compound aiding in digestion via the emulsification of lipids.

A human liver normally weighs between three to four pounds, and it is both the heaviest internal organ and the largest gland in the human body.

Non-alcoholic fatty liver disease is mainly found in developed countries; where a sedentary lifestyle and intake of high calories, high fat and high sugar are observed. It is the most common liver disorder worldwide and in the U.S.; about 30% of the U.S. population have NAFLD. NAFLD can also be found in children and adolescents because of growing obesity rate among children and adolescents. In NAFLD, you see accumulation of excess fat in liver cells up to 10 percent of the entire organ. Up to 65% of diabetic people have NAFLD without even knowing it, unless they are checked by their physicians, according to a study published in 2016 by the researchers at the University of California, San Diego. So, if you have diabetes, make sure your doctors check you for NAFLD.

NAFLD is asymptomatic, meaning it has no physical symptoms. Typically, excessive consumption of alcohol is a primary cause of fat build-up in the liver, but those with NAFLD may not drink at all or are moderate drinkers. The diagnosis of NAFLD can be done with blood tests, abdominal ultrasound and MRI, or a liver biopsy. NAFLD can progress to non-alcoholic steatohepatitis, cirrhosis (irreversible scarring of the liver with failure, or liver cancer. The medical community and public health officials project that obesity-related liver disease (cirrhosis and liver cancer) will become the leading cause of liver failure and liver transplantation in the near future.

Losing excess weight and maintaining healthy weight with balanced diet is the cornerstone of treatment along with regular exercise. Unfortunately, this is no easy task in our society dominated by a sedentary lifestyle and high-calorie, high-sugar and high-fat diet.

When you have elevated levels of blood triglycerides or LDL cholesterol, this can signal that there is too much fat in your liver. Your liver makes cholesterol on its own and circulates it into your blood stream. When you eat foods high in saturated and trans fats, the liver releases more fat and increases cholesterol levels.

According to German researchers analyzing over 3,000 participants, they found that those with NAFLD were three times more likely to have hypertension than those who did not have NAFLD.

If your family member has fatty liver disease, your risk of having NAFLD is at least 10 times higher, according to some studies that have shown that some people may be genetically predisposed to NAFLD.

You may experience some confusion at times since your liver is unable to metabolize properly with the toxins moving into the brain.

Besides excess alcohol, other things that can damage your liver include added sugar such as high-fructose corn syrup, some herbal supplements like kava kava taken by some women for post-menopausal symptoms, excessive drinking of soda, acetaminophen exceeding the recommended daily limits, vitamin A supplement in excess, and trans fats in some processed and packaged foods and baked goods.

It is important for you to nurture this amazing organ to ensure its optimal functioning for good health. The following is a list of foods that will help boost your liver functions to avoid or minimize hepatic damage:

- Water. People tend to take it for granted and the important role of water in health maintenance is often overlooked. Other than oxygen, your body needs water more than any other substances, including food, just to survive. It flushes toxins and waste products from your body, acting as an assistant to your liver. Instead of drinking sweet beverages like soda, you will be much better off switching to the ' plain old ' water, which keeps you hydrated and feeling full, a natural appetite suppressant.

⚕ Avocados. They are a great source of mono-unsaturated fatty acids; the fruit also contains glutathione, a nutrient for liver health.

⚕ Cruciferous vegetables. These dark leafy greens, including broccoli, kale, bok choy, daikon, and cauliflower, contain important phytonutrients --- flavonoids, carotenoids, sulforphane, and indoles --- to help your liver neutralize harmful chemicals, pesticides, drugs and carcinogens. In other words, these vegetables support your liver in its detoxification processes.

⚕ Sea vegetables. They help the liver detoxify your body by preventing assimilation of heavy metals as well as environmental toxins.

⚕ Eggs. They are an inexpensive source of high quality protein with all the eight essential amino acids for your liver to perform its detoxification processes optimally.

⚕ Garlic. It is an ancient land-based medicinal food, and contains an active sulfur-based compound called allicin, which plays a critical supportive role of liver detoxification. It helps the liver rid your body of mercury, certain food additives, and the hormone estrogen.

⚕ Onions, shallots and leeks. They are in the same family of garlic, containing sulfur compounds that support your liver in its production of glutathione, which helps neutralize free radicals.

- Artichokes. They contain two phytonutrients, cynarin and silymarin, which nourish your liver to promote the production of bile and help prevent formation of gall stones.

- Berries. They include strawberries, raspberries, blueberries and cranberries, all of them are rich in antioxidants. Their beneficial phytochemicals help your liver protect your body from free radicals and oxidative stress. Anthocyanins and polyphenols found in berries have been shown to inhibit growth of cancer cells in the liver, according to many studies.

- Apples. Eating an apple a day may just help to keep your doctor away. Like berries, apples contain polyphenols such as flavonoids which are anti-inflammatory. They also contain soluble fiber, pectin, that can help decrease toxic buildup in the body, making the job easier for your liver.

- Mushrooms. They are humble but powerful; the common ones include Shiitake, maitake and reishi. They contain nutrients which are important to support your immune system. One of their powerful antioxidants, L-eryothioeine, help liver neutralize the free radicals which are your cellular enemies.

- Coconut oil. Its healthy saturated fat is easy to digest in your saliva and gastric juices, meaning that your body does not need to make fat-digesting enzymes, which places less strain on your liver.

- Kimchi. This traditional Korean dish is made of fermented cabbage, radish, garlic, red pepper, onion, ginger and salt. Fermentation is an ancient form of preservation in which food is naturally transformed by microorganisms, breaking down carbohydrates and protein and aiding the digestive process.

- Ginger. This special spice has antioxidants which are anti-viral, anti-microbial and anti-inflammatory, supporting the detoxification process by the liver. Its other health benefits include improvement of circulation and unclogging of blocked arteries.

- Cardamom. It is part of the ginger family with important digestive role. It stimulates the flow of bile to improve fat metabolism.

- Turmeric. The curcumin compounds in turmeric, according to some studies, can help heal the liver and aid in its detoxification efforts.

- Coriander. Its seeds have been shown to aid the liver in lowering blood lipid levels among those with obesity and diabetes. They decrease triglyceride and LDL cholesterol levels while increasing HDL cholesterol. Its leaves, known as cilantro, help remove heavy metals from the body such as mercury and lead.

- Cumin. This is a flowering plant, native to the Mediterranean; it has long been considered a traditional medicinal herb. This spice has a number of potential health benefits; its antioxidants help protect your cells against oxidative stress caused by free radicals. In one Indian study, cumin was shown to boost the liver's detoxification power by stimulating the secretion of enzymes from the pancreas which helps your body to absorb nutrients.

Your liver is too important for you to ignore; once the damage is done with cirrhosis, it is permanent and irreversible. You can protect your liver by losing excess weight, especially the belly fat, with regular exercise, a plant-based diet, healthy lifestyle and a clean environment.

CHAPTER TWELVE

Bad foods to avoid

If you are considering taking excess body weight off, it is a good start. Overweight and obesity is a serious matter because your life and health are at stake. You must look at the big picture and start with one stroke at a time. Any ounce or pound lost is a step forward; even if you can only shed one pound a week, which is not difficult, you will have lost 52 pounds in one year. The name of this game is persistence, consistency and perseverance, finding something you can stick with, not the so-called ' crash diet '.

Remember that one famous saying: you are what you eat. So, first and foremost, learn and try to avoid certain foods, or at least cut them down as much as you can if you are serious about weight loss. We all have the experience of caving in to our cravings for certain favorite snacks and food every now and then, don't feel bad about it and be miserable. Just exercise your discipline, enjoy it with portion control and move on.

Many bad foods have serious health consequences, and if you can do your best to stay away from them, you will be way ahead on the road to a healthy, happy, meaningful life! There are quite a few unhealthy foods which are common in our American diet every day; some of the ' bad ' ingredients are hidden or inconspicuous and you have to be more mindful and vigilant before putting them into your body. The following list is not meant to be all inclusive, just to remind you and bring your attention to some of the common ones.

Processed meats.

These include sausages and hot dogs; in general, they represent a collection of meat that would otherwise be thrown away. These are combined with other products and chemicals to create artificially a palatable mixture of food. Processed meats often have high levels of salt, sodium, which not good for people who are trying to lose weight. They are also full of unhealthy fat and cholesterol with little nutritional value. The high sodium content can worsen existing high blood pressure, or an enlarged heart. If you have congestive heart failure or kidney disease or cirrhosis, the extra salt can contribute to a dangerous buildup of body fluid.

In fact, the World Health Organization in 2015 stated that processed meats are as bad as cigarette smoking regarding carcinogen content. They placed hot dogs, sausages and other processed meats in the same category of cancer risk as asbestos, alcohol, arsenic and tobacco.

In a recent study by the Harvard School of Public Health, people eating sausages and hot dogs have an increased risk of diabetes by 19%. The American Institute of Cancer Research supported these findings in 2015.

Bacon.

Bad news for the bacon lovers. Most of the bacon's calories come from fat, with almost half of that being the saturated variety.

Saturated fats are known to contribute to weight gain and increase the risk of heart disease and stroke. Saturated fats can also cause inflammation that accelerates skin aging with premature wrinkles. Bacon also contains sodium nitrate, as in other processed meats; sodium nitrate enhances oxidative stress according to a 2013 study published in the Journal of European Cytokine Network.

Fast foods.

Colloquially, we often call fast foods junk foods, and I think it is very appropriate to call them that. Fast foods typically are quick, calorific and fattening, containing a lot of sodium, unhealthy fat and added sugar. They are certainly a recipe for overweight and obesity, leading to heart disease, hypertension, high cholesterol and diabetes over time. The high salt content of fast foods can cause your bones to weaken because of sodium replacing the calcium, increasing your risk of osteoporosis.

Barbecued meats.

While everyone loves a good barbecue, grilling meats, besides their dripping, unhealthy fats, can produce carcinogens when the meats become charred. The two most carcinogens associated with charring are heterocyclic amines (HCA) and polycyclic aromatic hydrocarbon (PAH). Both are usually found when meat is cooked at high temperatures.

Potato Chips.

Everybody, young and old, loves potato chips. They are crispy and tasty, and they come in different flavors for your taste buds. Please be reminded that they have many calories, much fat and unhealthy amount of salt. These three things in potato chips make a terrible, perilous combination for anyone serious about weight loss. In a study of the New England Journal of Medicine in 2011, it was found that the link between weight gain and potato chips was stronger compared to other factors that caused weight gain like sugary beverages and processed meats. One serving, which is about 15 to 20 pieces, contains at least 154 calories and 10 grams of fat. The fats are mostly trans fats which stimulate interleukin-6 within your body to increase inflammation.

French fries.

French fries are one of the guiltiest pleasures, and one of the quickest ways to make you overweight in a short time. A small serving of French fries from popular fast food chains has an average of 200 to 330 calories. But with the growing popularity of supersized fries, you can have up to 700 calories for a large serving! When you go to have some fast food next time, it is advisable to skip the fries to avoid unintended sabotage to your weight loss efforts.

Fried foods.

These include chickens and fish all around you at the fast food establishments including regular restaurants. Fried foods contain trans fat and saturated fat with many calories per serving. If you continue to include them in your diet, you are bound to develop plaques in your arteries that will lead to heart attack and stroke. Many studies have already shown a definite link between saturated fat and arterial clogging, increasing the risk of stroke, heart attack and death considerably.

In 2013, a study published in the Nutrition, Metabolism and Cardiovascular Disease shows that eating fried foods more than four times a week increases the risk for obesity significantly compared to eating them just two times or less weekly. It is definitely a wise and healthy decision for you to cut down on fried foods, or eliminate them completely from your diet if you can in your weight loss journey.

Pizzas.

This is another popular food in our American culture. People love it even though they know it is unhealthy for the most part. You will be surprised by the extent of unhealthiness with eating pizza two to three times a week. One slice of pizza, in general, can contain up to 500 calories and 10 grams of saturated fat, and the numbers get even higher if you make it deep dish. Once you start adding cholesterol-laden toppings like sausages and pepperoni, the unhealthiness factor gets out of control. If you want to eat pizza once in a while, stick with the thin crust if you are doing the ordering, and you may want to use the opportunity to add some vegetables as toppings instead of sausages and pepperoni to offset the fattening effects of other ingredients in pizzas.

Instant noodles and soup.

They are quick and convenient, favorites for many homes and college campuses. Many of these instant noodles and soup contain excess salt, mono-sodium glutamate (the infamous MSG), added colors and flavors. They have very little nutritional value. MSG, according to some studies, can trigger migraine, in addition to some of its adverse health effects.

In fact, Baylor University researchers recently found that eating instant noodles two or more times a week raises your risk of metabolic syndrome, cardiovascular disease, stroke and diabetes. If you have a convenient need for instant noodles sometimes, you can add some nutrients to the noodles by including slices of broccoli and/or baby carrots, and ditching the soup after eating because most of the sodium is contained in the small package of soup base.

Ice cream

This popular dessert is everywhere, ubiquitous and pervasive in the American culture. Young and old, we all love it, and our taste buds are yearning for it. Very few of us want to admit that ice cream is bad; I think it is kind of a denial thing.

This delightful, likable dessert should be a concern for your health and weight if you eat it every day, or on a regular basis, say, two to three times a week or more. Ice cream, typically, is full of fat and cholesterol mixed with loads of sugar. It calls for a high fat content to make ice cream, at least 10% or more. In fact, some varieties can have up to 16%, and milk fat is mostly saturated fat. To make the health situation worse, some ice cream may contain some artificial sweeteners. Some studies have suggested that some artificial sweeteners promote overweight and obesity, and increase the risk of some types of cancer.

Baked goods

If you are in the process of losing weight or trying to lose wright, stay away from the bakery cases at the grocery stores. Baked goods are often rich in added sugar and fat, which can lead to weight gain. Sugar, in excess, can promote an unhealthy microbiome in your gut and it can also cause inflammation for your body. Look at the baked goods as an occasional treats, not a regular things to eat.

Packaged cakes and cookies

They typically contain trans fat, which is partially hydrogenated oil to keep the food shelf-stable and moist. A lot of preservatives are also added to prevent spoiling. These sweet, palatable things are unhealthy and fattening, and it is prudent and wise to avoid them, or cut down on their consumption as part of your weight loss program.

Cheese

It is the biggest offender in pizzas. Cheese is incredibly dense, and is packed with solid milk fat which is very high in cholesterol and calories. Despite its other nutritional value, this high-calorie food has an average of 100 calories per ounce. Eating too much of it in a day or pair it with other foods rich in calories and you will be closer to weight gain than you will be to weight loss.

According to the United States Department of Agriculture, the average American eats about 30 pounds of cheese every year which is three times more than the amount they consumed 40 years ago.

Coupled with its relatively high sodium content, consumption of cheese without moderation can lead to overweight and obesity, hypertension, hyperlipidemia and cardiovascular disease.

Biscuits and gravy

Biscuits are usually made with refined flour and shortening, a major source of trans fat, in order to make them light and flaky. The gravy is essentially fat, then milk or cream is added. This combination is one of the unhealthiest foods man has ever made. Its consumption is a sure obstacle in your road to healthy weight.

Frozen TV dinners

They might be convenient. Very few of them have anything to offer in the ways of nutritional value. Many people do not realize that these so-called TV dinners are processed foods. They are usually full of fat, calories and sodium in order to make something that has just been microwaved palatable after sitting in a freezer for months. TV dinners that are low in fat are also unhealthy, even though advertisements might tell you otherwise; they are still highly processed, and full of chemicals and sodium.

Margarine

There was a short time when it was believed that margarine was healthier than butter, but that has gone out the window. It is often made with partially hydrogenated oil, one of the most common trans fats harmful to your heart and arteries. Use a healthier fat like olive oil, or just stick with a small amount of real butter.

Pasta

Pasta is rich in carbohydrates with a high glycemic index. This means that as soon as it is digested, your blood sugar levels will spike. A pasta dish with cheese and meats cooked in oil definitely increases the calorie count significantly with much unhealthy fats, impeding weight loss.

Soda and diet soda

These beverages including energy drinks are toxic sugars in disguise. Soda and diet soda are very inexpensive; you can buy a case of 24 – 12oz cans for about four dollars and up to eight to nine dollars, depending on the brands and time of sale.

Almost all nutritionists and dieticians advise people to avoid soda and sugary drinks completely. Soda can become an addiction for some people, similar to tobacco, alcohol and drugs; it may feel good when you drink it, it can wreak havoc on your body long-term.

Many researchers have shown that these sugary beverages including the diet ones are directly linked to weight gain and all other diseases, from type-2 diabetes, heart disease and hypertension to cancer, dementia and infertility.

Diet soda tastes the same as regular soda because they have artificial sweeteners. These artificial sweeteners play tricks on the brain, which thinks the body is consuming more calories than it actually is, eventually leading to appetite problems. In the end, people end up eating more. Another problem with artificial sweeteners in diet soda is changing the gut microbes, increasing the risk of type-2 diabetes due to insulin resistance.

In a study conducted by the University of Texas Health Science Center at San Antonio, people who drank two or more diet soda a day had waist sizes that were six times bigger than those who did not drink diet soda. The study was conducted on over 470 participants for a period of ten years.

I can't think of anything good about drinking soda including diet soda. It is an addiction, similar to alcohol and drugs because it feels good when you drink it, but it can wreak havoc on your body long-term.

One of the easiest ways to lose weight is to cut soda from your diet. If you are drinking it several times a day, say, three to four cans, cutting down to one to two cans a day could be a good start until you are eventually comfortable with just one or two cans a week or eliminating it completely from your diet. According to one study by weight loss experts, dropping a daily large Coca Cola from fast food joints completely would result in reducing your annual calorie intake by 200,000 calories --- or about 60 pounds --- in one year! So, if you are a rabid soda drinker and motivated to lose weight, this is one easy way to overcome obesity.

Popcorns at movie theaters

Plain popcorn is a healthy grain, but when it is eaten at the movie theaters is a totally different story. The corns are usually loaded with unhealthy fats, added sugar and lots of salt in a big bucket. Try to resist it and focus on the movie you are going to enjoy. Sitting still for two hours and piling on all that calories will certainly ruin your weight loss plan.

Bagels

Bagels are made with refined white flour, which has had all of its nutritional value processed out of it. Bagels are very dense, in some cases, the equivalent of eating six slices of bread. Each contains an average of 400 calories with a high glycemic index, which promotes insulin resistance and increases inflammation within your body. When you add the butter and cream cheese, you will bring back some of the pounds lost.

Cinnabon

They are so unhealthy that they are in a class all by themselves. A classic cinnabon contains at least 800 calories and 38 grams of fat, half of which are saturated. They are also loaded with sugar to enhance your taste. If you are serious about losing excess weight, do not get anywhere near them.

Toaster pastries

They are convenient things to eat in the morning, but unhealthy in the long run when you look at them more closely. The crust is made with white, refined flour and unhealthy fat; the filling and icing is mostly sugar. Having it for breakfast once in a while may be acceptable; make yourself a hard-boiled egg instead, three to times a week and it will keep you full before lunch without sugar spikes and crashes.

Pancakes

They are a good source of carbohydrates and proteins, and contain a wide range of vitamins and minerals. When you top them off with saturated fats (butter), sugars (the so-called maple syrup) and salt, they become unhealthy breakfast. If you have a taste for them once in a while, ask for honey instead of syrup and be easy on the butter.

Fruit drinks.

These seemingly healthy fruit drinks from restaurants and fast food chains contain, in addition to other additives, certain amount of added sugar, usually fructose, the type associated with the development of visceral adipose tissue --- that is belly fat. You are much better off drinking the juice from fresh fruits.

Candies

There are so many different varieties to suit just about everyone's taste. Unfortunately, they usually have harmful ingredients including artificial coloring, added sugar and saturated fats.

Chinese food from carryout

They are often loaded with MSG, monosodium glutamate, a flavor and appetite enhancer which causes you to gain weight, in addition to the added sugar and unhealthy fats. If you have a craving for Chinese food once in a while, make sure it is MSG-free and resist the soy sauce that comes with your food.

Doritos

One of its harmful ingredients is MSG. The powerful savory taste also lingers in your mouth after eating, a tactic called ' long hang-time flavor ' to lure snackers to go back for more. If you are serious about weight loss, try to do without them to make the battle easier.

Cheetos

They are typically doused with MSG, in addition to other additives. Food developers know that when foods melt quickly inside your mouth, it tricks the brain into thinking you are not eating as many calories and need more.

Oreos

Their ingredients include palm oil, processed cocoa and high fructose corn syrup, all of which are not exactly healthy. Palm oil is a fat that promotes fat-causing inflammation. According to some studies in 2013, cookies are one of the most difficult to eat in moderation. If you have a craving for a cookie treat, exercise portion control as much as you can.

Commercially packed muffins

They contain ingredients such as soybean oil, high fructose corn syrup, and trans fats, and they are not the ingredients you want to eat for weight loss. One innocent –looking muffin like blueberry muffin can carry up to 400 calories, and many people can consume more than one as snack!

Many of the foods described above often lack in fiber, protein, and nutrients that help nourish you and fill you up, thus leading you to overeating.

In summary, you should avoid or keep to a minimum the following list of foods for the sake of healthy eating and healthy weight:

- Added sugars. They contain almost no nutrients and are pure carbohydrates with empty calories.

- Dairy fat. This includes ice cream, whole milk and cheese products, which are usually full of saturated fat and some naturally occurring trans fat.

- White carbohydrates. These include bread, pasta, rice, cookies, cakes and pancakes. If you like them, switch to the whole-grain versions.

- Baked sweets. The commercially prepared versions are generally packed with processed carbohydrates,, added sugars, unhealthy fat and salt.

- Processed and high-fat meats. They can be found just about everywhere, and they include bacon, ham, pepperoni, hot dogs and many lunch meat. Their proteins are less healthy than the proteins from fish, skinless chicken, nuts, beans, and whole grains. Fresh red meat should be consumed sparingly and the leanest cut selected.

- Salt. Current dietary guidelines and the American Heart Association recommend up to 1,500 mg of sodium per day and not to exceed 2,300 mg of total sodium intake per day. Most of the people consume about one and a half teaspoons of salt daily, translating to about 3,400 mg of sodium and increasing the risk of high blood pressure, stroke, heart disease and obesity.

CLOSING SUMMARY

It is very important to set realistic goals for yourself to avoid falling off the weight-loss wagon. More often than not, people who have set unrealistic goals, whether weight loss or something else, tend to throw in the towel for good when as though they have failed.

After your reading of this book, you have already learnt that there are many ways and foods that can help you lose excess weight and maintain your healthy weight. Dropping pounds is a great long-term goal, not a sprint. Instead of taking on a heavy load off, focus on just losing a pound a week. Even with losing one pound a week, which is not difficult or insurmountable, that is 52 pounds a year. You will be surprised how small tweaks can result in major change without stress.

Severely restricting your calorie intake, like eating 1,000 calories a day or less, may lead to some weight loss temporarily, but you will gain it all back plus more as soon as you start eating normally again, not to mention that starving yourself can be dangerous!

Please be reminded that the " all or none " strategy of weight loss will ultimately fail. Cutting out indulgences may sound good and may help you lose weight, but over time, it will make you feel deprived and eventually lead to bingeing. It is better to reward yourself once in a while with your cravings so that you can stay on track, as long as you exercise your portion control. Remind yourself to pay attention to your internal hunger/satiety cues to determine whether you really want or need that second chocolate chip cookie or not, and not just rely on what other people around you are eating or seductive advertising.

Don't abuse your body including your brain by skimping on sleep because you will be more susceptible to weight gain, thus, unconsciously sabotaging your weight-loss efforts. This is well-proven scientifically by many studies: sleep-deprived people tend to consume more calories daily than those who get a full night's rest of 7 to 8 hours.

Physical activities and exercise are crucial and should be part of your daily living, especially if you are trying to lose weight. There are many different types of physical activities as already mentioned in this book, either at home, at work, outside your home or office. If you decide to pursue an exercise program which is very commendable, start and progress slowly and gradually to avoid potential injury and excessive soreness that may prevent or deter you from sticking to your exercise program.

I do not advise micro-managing down to the level of every gram of everything you eat; the overall awareness and mindfulness tends to create the most success long term.

If you are feeling stuck on the plateau, try some High Intensity Interval Training, HIIT, to torch your calories with a jolt in as few as 10 to 15 minutes a day. Here, when you boost your muscle mass with HIIT, you will increase your fat-burning potential all day long. Do not beat yourself up if you mess up or slip sometimes; consistency is the key, and don't let one bad day turn into a bad week. Do not get discouraged; positive mental attitude is crucial for lasting weight loss.

Stay with a plant-based diet, with 80% of your food intake consisting of fruit and vegetables. Socialize with friends who have the same healthy goals you are pursuing and maintain a healthy lifestyle. You will find losing weight and keeping healthy weight a possible and enjoyable endeavor.

Good health and good luck!

www.ingramcontent.com/pod-product-compliance
Lightning Source LLC
Chambersburg PA
CBHW020511290526
45786CB00002B/558